Springer Series on Child and Family Studies

Series Editor

Nirbhay N. Singh, Medical College of Georgia, Augusta University, Augusta, GA, USA

The Springer Series on Child and Family Studies addresses fundamental psychological, educational, social, and related issues within the context of child and family research. Volumes published in this series examine clinical topics with an additional focus on epidemiological, developmental, and life span issues. Leading scholars explore such factors as race and immigration, parenting, and the effects of war and violence on military families and unite a vast literature into a comprehensive series of related research volumes.

Laura Nabors · Tina L. Stanton-Chapman
Editors

Developmental Disabilities and Chronic Illness in Young Children

Promoting Positive Development and Outcomes

Springer

Editors
Laura Nabors
School of Human Services
University of Cincinnati
Cincinnati, OH, USA

Tina L. Stanton-Chapman
Early Childhood Education and Human Development
University of Cincinnati
Cincinnati, OH, USA

ISSN 2570-0421 ISSN 2570-043X (electronic)
Springer Series on Child and Family Studies
ISBN 978-3-032-08522-1 ISBN 978-3-032-08523-8 (eBook)
https://doi.org/10.1007/978-3-032-08523-8

This Springer imprint is published by the registered company Springer Nature Switzerland AG
The registered company address is: Gewerbestrasse 11, 6330 Cham, Switzerland

Preface

Developmental Disabilities and Chronic Illness in Young Children: Promoting Positive Development and Outcomes was developed to provide information to promote well-being for young children with developmental disabilities or illnesses, who would benefit from support to promote their well-being across different contexts. Positive outcomes in different settings that are critical for children, such as school and extracurricular activities are discussed, in the hopes of providing information that will enhance positive development in children's everyday lives. This will provide knowledge to health professionals assisting children and families, to promote resilience in the context of child and family life. Promoting resilience in contexts of daily life is an approach to wellness that has the potential to meet children and families where they are, which is consistent with a child- and family-centered approach to wellness that has the potential to promote child and family resilience and child emotional, social, and physical wellness as well as academic achievement and positive functioning in key settings for the child and family. Meeting children and families where they are and with day-to-day needs can help address health disparities, because a child- and family-oriented approach where help is needed may mean provision of additional "supports," and this can be interventions, adjusting environments, or adding support services, for those that need them. Chapters focus on review of the evidence base and interventions to promote positive functioning in children and emphasize a systems-based approach to ensure that supports surround the child and family—in order to promote positive developmental trajectories. As such, the purpose of this book is to be a resource or tool kit with information for professionals and clinicians working with children with developmental disabilities and chronic illnesses to attenuate risk factors and promote resilience, using interventions that work, in the context of children's everyday lives.

Cincinnati, OH, USA

Laura Nabors
Tina L. Stanton-Chapman

Contents

Chapter 1
Children with Developmental Disabilities and Chronic Illnesses

Laura Nabors and Tina L. Stanton-Chapman

Abstract This chapter synthesizes evidence on the prevalence, impacts, and educational inclusion of children with chronic illnesses and developmental disabilities in preschool and elementary years. It documents variable but rising prevalence (with some severe conditions), frequent mental health comorbidity, and disparities by sex and race/ethnicity. While educational support services show mental health benefits, evidence for academic gains remains mixed, particularly for younger children. The chapter advances Response to Intervention and Universal Design for Learning as complementary frameworks to identify needs early, reduce barriers, and deliver tiered, accessible supports. It highlights implementation variability across states, dependence on educator training, and gaps in progress monitoring. Community- and family-centered interventions demonstrate improved caregiver self-efficacy, child quality of life, and family integration, including promising digital and simulation-based approaches. Priorities include stronger causal evidence for early academic outcomes, equity-focused research, and coordinated school–healthcare–family systems to promote inclusion and optimize developmental trajectories.

Keywords Prevalence · Chronic illnesses · Developmental disabilities; educational support; response to intervention · Universal design · Family-centered interventions

---

L. Nabors (✉)
School of Human Services, College of Education, Criminal Justice, Human Services, and Information Technology, University of Cincinnati, Cincinnati, OH, USA
e-mail: naborsla@ucmail.uc.edu

T. L. Stanton-Chapman
Early Childhood Education and Human Development, School of Education, College of Education, Criminal Justice, Human Services, and Information Technology, University of Cincinnati, Cincinnati, OH, USA

L. Nabors and T. Stanton-Chapman (eds.), *Developmental Disabilities and Chronic Illness in Young Children*, Springer Series on Child and Family Studies,
https://doi.org/10.1007/978-3-032-08523-8_1

Prevalence Chronic Illnesses

Chronic illnesses or health conditions are defined in many ways, with one hallmark feature being they are often non-communicable diseases, and within a broad conceptualization of chronic illnesses prevalence rates can be as high as 44% of children (Barnett et al., 2023). In another study, van der Lee et al. (2007) reported a prevalence rate from 22% to 44%. A smaller percentage (around 5%) may have serious conditions (Barnett et al., 2023; Newacheck & Taylor, 1992). About one in four children has a chronic condition, although prevalence rates vary based on the type of chronic illness, and whether the sample is focused on one type of illness (e.g., diabetes only) or many types of illnesses, and the severity of the conditions for the children (Barrio Cortes et al., 2020). Chronic health conditions in children have demonstrated an increasing trend (Hall et al., 2019; Perrin et al., 2007), with about 7% of children with these conditions facing limitations and approximately 1–2% of these youth receiving disability benefits for their medical issues (Perrin et al., 2007). Children with chronic illnesses face risk for developing mental health problems (Delamater et al., 2017). Morgan (2019) reported that anywhere from about ten percent to over one-third of children with chronic illnesses can develop mental health problems (e.g., anxiety, depression), which is a higher level of these problems compared to children in the general population. Some have mentioned that having chronic conditions place children at greater risk for experiencing child maltreatment (Jaudes, & Mackey-Bilaver, 2008).

Although the severity of impact of an illness may be greater for older children (Newacheck & Halfon, 1998), chances for positively impacting child development may be greater when intervening with young children, and this sets an early pattern of success for families. Prevalence rates vary for young children. For instance, Blackwell et al. (2019) assessed parent report of chronic illnesses for 1253 children between the ages of 5–9 years (mean age of about 6 years) and found that about 20% of the children in their sample had one chronic health problem, while about 8.5% had two or more health problems. Most of their sample was white; however, they did assess families across an array of income levels (Blackwell et al., 2019). It may be that their rates were lower, because they focused on younger children, but this study is another example of the varying rates of chronic illnesses across studies. Interestingly, although the young children with chronic illnesses had poorer health than children without health conditions, life satisfaction of children did not differ based on whether the child had or did not have a chronic illness. We realize that children's chronic illnesses may have comorbid developmental disabilities (and vice versa), but we present each separately to highlight the importance of each type of healthcare condition.

Prevalence of Developmental Disabilities

In education, students with developmental disabilities are those children who require special education and/or related services to be successful in the school environment (Hallahan et al., 2024). The Individuals with Disabilities Education Act (IDEA) is the special education law that determines who does and does not qualify for special education and related services. Specifically, IDEA indicates that a student qualifies for special education and/or related services if they: (a) meet a minimum of one or more of the 13 eligible disability categories (e.g., specific learning disability, speech or language impairment, other health impairment, autism, intellectual disability, emotional disturbance, developmental delay, multiple disabilities, hearing impairment, orthopedic impairment, visual impairment, traumatic brain injury, deaf-blindness) and (b) the disability adversely affects the student's educational performance in school (U.S. Department of Education, 2004). Eligibility is determined through a thorough evaluation of the student's abilities and the student's age—ages three through 21 years. According to the 2019–2021 National Health Interview Survey (NHIS, U.S. Department of Health and Human Services, 2023), the prevalence of developmental disabilities in children aged 3–17 years increased from 7.40% (2019) to 8.56% (2021) for a total of 7.5 million children receiving school-based special education services under IDEA. Taken as a percentage of total public-school enrollment, this equates to 15% of students (National Center for Education Statistics, 2024). Specific learning disabilities, speech or language impairments, other health impairments, and autism were the most frequent categories represented by students with Individual Education Plans (IEPs) (U.S. Department of Education Statistics, 2024).

More male students (18%) than female students (10%) were serviced under IDEA (National Center for Education Statistics, 2024). Female students were more likely to be identified with learning disabilities (42%) whereas male students were more likely to be identified with autism (16%). By race and ethnicity, the percentage of public-school students served under IDEA in 2022–2023 was: American Indian/Alaska Native (19%), Black (17%), White (16%), two or more races (16%), Hispanic (15%), Pacific Islander (12%), and Asian (8%) (National Center for Education Statistics, 2024). Sixty percent of these students spent the majority of their day in the general education classroom with typical peers.

Critical Nature of Educational Support

In their review of four educational support interventions (three included children with cancer and one for children with ADHD), Barnett et al. (2023) noted mixed results in terms of a positive impact on academic achievement. They did report that educational interventions were supportive of the mental health needs of children. However, the age ranges of children participating in the studies varied (typically it was about

6 years and older, but the age range in studies was 4–18 years), and it was difficult to determine the specific impact of interventions for elementary schoolers. And, information on the educational support needs of preschoolers and very young children were not accounted for. Moreover, Barnett et al. (2023) indicated that improving understanding of educational needs for children with chronic illnesses is a direction for future research.

Developing Interventions and Planning for Inclusion at School

Given the critical nature of educational support, we recommend Response to Intervention (RTI) as one starting point for assisting young children with chronic illnesses and developmental disabilities in school settings. Moreover, universal design, which can ensure that all spaces are inclusive and welcoming of children with special healthcare needs (e.g., being in a wheelchair) is beneficial to child development. We describe RTI in the next section of this chapter, followed by a section on universal design (UD), as both are methods to promote the development and inclusion of children with chronic illnesses and developmental disabilities. Although we present critique of UD or the universal design learning approach, we propose that combined with RTI it has merit for ensuring that the design of spaces is conducive to the inclusion of children with chronic illnesses and developmental disabilities.

Response to Intervention (RTI)

IDEA (2004) incorporated the Response to Intervention (RTI) strategy as an alternative process for identifying students with disabilities, specifically learning disabilities (Individuals with Disabilities Education Improvement Act of 2004, 2004). We believe this approach can facilitate inclusion of children with all types of special healthcare needs, including the myriad of chronic illnesses and developmental disabilities. RTI is a tiered intervention which provides research-supported effective instruction that is based on a student's needs (Aspiranti et al., 2019). The RTI framework includes three tiers of instruction. Tier 1 instruction is received by all students. Students are typically administered a universal screener to collect baseline data that is used to identify students who need additional instructional support (Hogan, 2024). The overall goal of the universal screener is to comprehend how each student is performing on academic standards and content. Students who successfully pass the screener remain in Tier 1 instruction while students who do not successfully pass the screener receive Tier 2 instruction.

Tier 2 intervention typically includes evidence-based small group guided skills practice (Nilvius et al., 2021). Skills practice is typically defined in duration, frequency, and length of sessions of moderate intensity (i.e., 8-to-15 weeks of 20-to-40-min sessions) (National Center for Response to Intervention, 2010). Tier 2 interventions typically focus on academic and/or behavior intervention(s). An example of Tier 2 math intervention is the use of a graphic organizer which helps students organize and manage their problem-solving (e.g., what do I need to find out? what do I need to do to solve the problem? how I solved the problem? how I checked my answer?). After 6-to-8 weeks, Tier 2 students are reevaluated to determine growth (Hogan, 2024). If students make adequate progress, they return to Tier 1 instruction. If students have not made adequate progress, they remain in Tier 2 instruction.

Tier 3 intervention is the most intensive and is individualized to target each student's area of needs (National Center for Response to Intervention, 2010). Tier 3 intervention is typically provided in the general education classroom or as a pull-out service (Hogan, 2024). Teachers tend to begin with a more intensive intervention of what was provided in Tier 2. This may mean longer instructional sessions, and/or higher frequency of sessions. Further assessments reveal where the student is having difficulty in their academic learning and/or behavior. Once problematic areas are revealed, intense intervention begins. An example of an intense intervention is the *Copy, Cover,* and *Compare* strategy (Skinner, McLaughlin, & Logan, 1997). In this strategy, the student is given a worksheet containing math facts to practice. The student studies each math fact with the answer that appears on the sheet. The student then *covers* the fact and *copies* it from memory. The student then *compares* their copied math with the original correct model to check for accuracy. When a student is able to copy a fact with the answer from memory without errors three times, the fact is considered mastered (Joseph et al., 2011).

Across all RTI tiers, progress monitoring is a key component. Progress monitoring is the continuous and frequent collection of student data to: (a) assess students' performance and (b) quantify a student's rate of improvement or responsiveness to RTI intervention tiers (American Institutes for Research, 2025). Data from progress monitoring are used to determine if students need more intensive interventions, improved in their skill acquisition, and/or are in need of different instructional forms or styles. This information is then used to move students across the intervention tiers for instructional purposes.

As previously discussed, RTI is an alternate procedure for early identification of possible disabilities in preschoolers and school-age children. Studies examining the effectiveness of the RTI approach (e.g., Armendariz & Jung, 2016; Arias-Gundin & Llamazares, 2021) have indicated that the decision to use the RTI model is often made at the legislative level with little input from school administrators and teachers. Maki et al. (2018) reported that 16% of states require RTI as the single model of learning disability classification. The remaining states use a combination of methods. Berkeley et al. (2020) reported that 39 states encourage the use of tiers to support students with special needs, but do not necessarily require RTI as an identification mandate. Responsibility for interpreting and implementing RTI procedures falls on states and local school districts, and thus, there is significant variance within and across states (Hudson & McKenzie, 2016).

RTI success is ultimately dependent on the knowledge and preparedness of those who are responsible for implementation (Berkeley et al., 2020). As a whole, educators, while seeing the value in RTI, report a need for more training and support in the use of RTI particularly in the areas of data collection, data analysis, and how and when to move students between the tiers (Hogan, 2024). For progress monitoring purposes, a literature review of studies using the RTI approach in reading found that many educators only perform one evaluation at the beginning and one evaluation at the end of an intervention period in Tiers 1 and 2 (e.g., bimonthly, quarterly) (Arias-Gundin & Llamazares, 2021). These two tiers are typically implemented by general education teachers who may not have the specialized training needed to implement individual and small group interventions. Despite these findings, however, RTI has evidence of effectiveness.

Universal Design

With the reauthorization of IDEA in 2004, the term *universal design* (UD) was defined within federal law (Edyburn, 2010). Universal design was originally defined by architect, Ronald Mace, as a means to design physical spaces in a manner that promotes accessibility for individuals of all abilities. UD focuses on the physical environment and promotes access to buildings (e.g., elevators, ramps, entrances to the building), structured environments (e.g., sidewalks, parking spaces), public transportation (e.g., subways, busses, airplanes), and products (e.g., toilets, self-care) (Mace, 1998; Anastasiou et al., 2024). Rose and Meyer (2002) extended Mace's work and applied UD to education with the universal design for learning (UDL) approach.

UDL ideology centers on making the learning curriculum accessible to students of all ability levels rather than focusing on student deficits (Rose & Meyer, 2002). The UDL framework consists of three principles: (a) *multiple means of representation:* teachers present content in multiple, flexible ways to provide students several options to acquire, process, and integrate knowledge and information; (b) *multiple means of action and expression:* teachers provide multiple and flexible ways for students to demonstrate what they have learned; and (c) *multiple means of engagement:* teachers provide flexible options for students' interests, abilities, and motivation (Hall et al., 2012). These guidelines are further illustrated through two to five checkpoints which provide recommendations for designing learning experiences tailored to individual students (Zhang et al., 2024). Teachers use the guidelines to anticipate and reduce barriers to learning (Ok et al., 2017).

Unal et al. (2022) developed a UDL lesson plan template which can be used to develop UDL lesson plans. The lesson plan body is guided by four main components and corresponding questions. The first component is *input. Input* asks teachers, "which methods and techniques will you use to help students' learning?" and "how is this lesson connected to the students' prior knowledge?" The second component is *modeling. Modeling* asks teachers, "how will you help students in learning (e.g., verbal explanation, visual cues, demo lessons)?" The third component is *guided practice. Guided practice* asks teachers, "how will students practice their skills?" and "what techniques will you use to provide guidance?" The fourth component is *unprompted practice. Unprompted practice* asks teachers, "how will students demonstrate skill independently?"

The following illustrates an UDL lesson plan using Unal et al. (2022)'s lesson plan template as guidance:

A second-grade teacher developed a UDL lesson plan for the standard, "Students will be able to identify the main elements of a story (i.e., characters, setting, plot)." Her students previously worked on identifying characters and settings in a story and writing sentences to show their understanding of these concepts. In this lesson, the teacher wished to add the plot element to the lesson plan and have students write their own story with one or more characters, a setting, and a clear plot. The teacher selected the book, Dear Max by Sally Grindly, for her lesson. Dear Max is about a boy named Max who receives a book for Christmas and he begins to write the author where the two parties begin a creative journey of creative writing with each helping the other write.

The teacher decided to use a variety of methods to teach the concept of plot. The first method to teach the concept of plot was whole-class implicit instruction. Whole-class implicit instruction centered on vocabulary development to define the terms: plot, beginning, middle, and end, a plot graphic organizer (see below), and the book, Three Little Pigs.

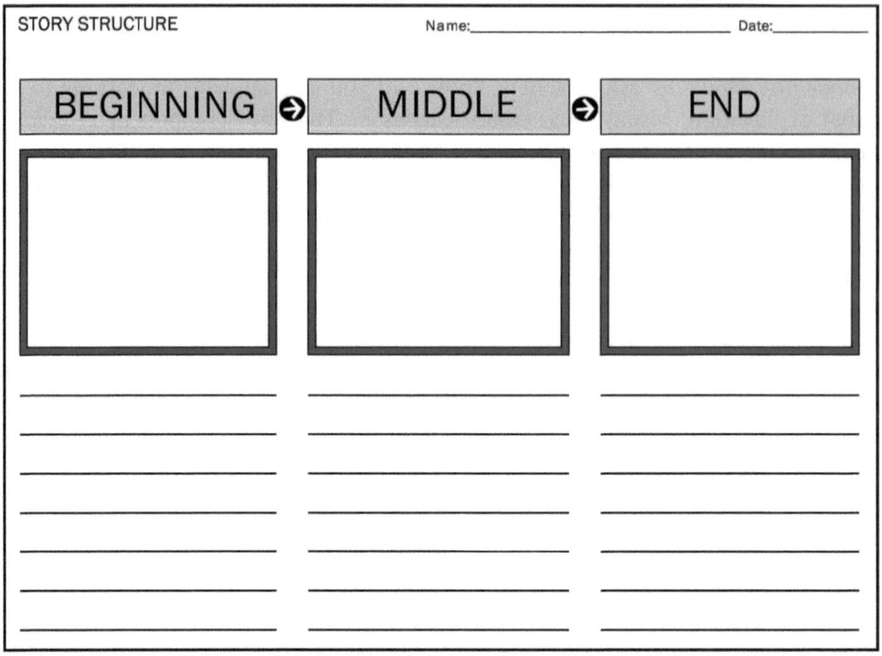

Students were familiar with the Three Little Pigs book from previous lessons. Each student had a printed copy of the book. As a class, the teacher walked the class through the process of how to identify the beginning, middle, and end plot elements using the graphic organizer and the book.

The second method to teach the concept of plot was group or individual work. Students had the choice of working in small groups or individually where they completed plot graphic organizers using various books. Students selected the books they wished to use for the lessons. Choices included audio books, printed copies of books, or books on video. If students had difficulty with the plot concept, the teacher had multiple means of assistance including one-to-one guidance with the teacher, printed resources describing plots, videos which explained a story's plot, and computer games on how to find a story's plot.

The third method to teach the concept of plot was the book, Dear Max. Students had several options for this portion of the lesson. They could read a printed copy of the book on their own. They could participate in a read-aloud of the book with the teacher. They could listen to an audio recording of the book. They could watch a video of the book. When the reading was completed, they independently completed a graphic organizer which asked them to provide details of the characters, the setting, and the plot. Students could demonstrate their understanding of Dear Max by drawing pictures, writing words, or writing a sentence or two in each box of the graphic organizer.

In the UDL lesson just described, students were given choices in their learning. The teacher did not determine their abilities through assessments as seen in the RTI approach. Students select how they wished to participate in the lesson (e.g., small group, individually) and the format of their learning (e.g., reading a book with the teacher, listening to an audio book, reading a printed copy of a book on their own, watching a video of the book). For the assessment phases of the lesson, students could draw pictures, write words, or write sentences to demonstrate their learning. The overall thought with this intervention approach is that the student rather than the teacher determines how they will best demonstrate their success within their given ability.

Prior research on UDL demonstrates not only support of UDL techniques from teachers, researchers, and policymakers, but evidence of its effectiveness in the classroom (Hollingshead et al., 2022). Studies have shown UDL's effectiveness in elementary and secondary education classrooms with students receiving special education services and in university settings (Fornauf & Erickson, 2020; Kennedy et al., 2013; Ok et al., 2017). UDL's use is also suggested in U.S. federal education policies (e.g., Every Student Succeeds Act of 2015) (Zhang et al., 2024).

Although UDL has evidence of research and policy support, the approach is not without criticism. The first criticism centers on whether UDL is based on a well-established theory (Anastasiou et al., 2024). Critics of UDL indicate that the developers of UDL oversimplified the cognitive processes involved in learning and do not account for the process of how children learn (Demetriou et al., 2024). In other words, they posit that UDL does not properly address working and long-term memory (Anastasiou et al., 2024). Both working and long-term memory play a critical role in learning and retaining information. Children with cognitive disabilities such as learning disabilities or cognitive disabilities (e.g., children with cancer experiencing late effects of the chemotherapy treatment) may have delays in their working and long-term memory which may impact their ability to learn (Bortfeld & Bunge, 2024).

A second criticism of UDL focuses on whether it is possible to meet the needs of all learners in a given classroom (Anastasiou et al., 2024). For example, Hitchcock et al. (2005) highlighted that it is nearly impossible to meet the needs of all students across the continuum and empirical evidence for UDL's effectiveness is based on ideas and assumptions that the approach is working. In other words, it is impossible to develop a lesson plan for everyone. Critics such as Hallahan et al. (2024) posit that many students with disabilities need specially designed instruction that includes implicit instruction, more frequent feedback, and individualized assistance. Some even question the need for Individualized Education Plans (IEPs) if UDL is as effective as the developers believe (Anastasiou et al., 2024).

A third criticism of UDL is the complexity of testing its effectiveness (Anastasiou et al., 2024). Edyburn (2010) argues that UDL is a framework that has multiple interpretations of what it looks like in practice. How one teacher interprets the UDL framework can be entirely different from how a different teacher interprets it. Interpretation variability impacts both validity and reliability (Zhang et al., 2024). In addition, studies that have researched the impact of UDL have not used comparison groups in their effectiveness test (AlRawi & Alkahtani, 2021). Although UDL has shortcomings, combined with an RTI approach, it can help with design and modification of learning environments to facilitate the inclusion of young children on playgrounds and in the classroom, which has the potential to support their academic, social, and emotional development.

Community-Based Interventions

Watkinson et al. (2023) conducted a systematic review focusing on evaluation of interventions in community settings (as well as some in homes) to improve care of children with multiple types of medical conditions, who might be considered medically fragile. Twenty-five articles (from 1999 to 2021) were reviewed. Children had different types of medical conditions, including developmental disabilities, and ranged in age from infancy to high school age (16 years). Interventions often targeted parents and could also be developed for extended family (grandparents), foster parents, or childcare providers or to include school staff. Interventions often were education-based, with either in-person individual or group experiences or information sent via email. Support groups also were a common intervention, and these could be combined with psycho-education sessions. Some internet-based or mobile health interventions also were reviewed. In terms of education, some of the interventions provided simulation activities, to better equip caregivers to handle medical emergencies for the child. Watkinson et al. (2023) reported that interventions had positive outcomes, leading to increased self-sufficiency in caring for the child on the part of caregivers. Improved quality of life for the child and increased feelings of self-efficacy and empowerment resulted for caregivers participating in interventions. Improving family-based care could lead to improved family integration in their community, with a return to more normal family routines. The authors concluded that more research for children in low-income families, who reside in disadvantaged communities, and more studies on improving inclusive education and developing a patient-centered medical home are needed, to continue to improve quality of life for children and families. This review was insightful; however, it was noteworthy that databases reviewed were more medically oriented and review of studies in psychologically-oriented databases might reveal other interventions.

Nur et al. (2023) conducted a systematic review and meta-analysis of family-focused, community-based interventions, including more psychology-oriented databases in their search for evidence-based interventions. Studies that incorporated randomized controlled trials were included in their review and the databases they used were assessed from dates of inception until 2022, and eight studies met review criteria. Three studies focused on education, four on relationships, and one study combined both approaches. In addition to finding that educationally oriented interventions improved family life, they also determined that relationship-based interventions strengthened child and family functioning and quality of life. They noted that role-play in interventions was a way to address stress, processing emotions, and facilitate coping. Results of improvement in family functioning were equivocal. Moreover, findings were equivocal for improvement in child symptoms, with some studies indicating improvement in disease-related symptoms, while others did not show improvement. It was encouraging that symptom improvement did occur in some studies (e.g., in three out of six studies that were reviewed asthma and diabetes symptoms improved) related to participating in family-based, supportive interventions. The researchers proposed that education alone might not be enough, and adding role play to review and practice the use of critical information might improve the messaging and uptake of educational information so that increased positive change could occur. Only one study assessed knowledge change as the result of the intervention, and change in knowledge was positive, indicating a positive impact of education about the disease and managing it. Seven of the studies were conducted in homes, with one being in a school setting, and therefore, information about long-term change was limited. Nur et al. (2023) recommended that future research be conducted in community settings and center on role-playing to enhance learning and also focus on techniques to improve family communication. Similar to Watkinson et al. (2023), Nur et al. recommended that research focusing on families residing in disadvantaged communities will provide important contributions to the field.

Family-Centered Interventions

Chow et al. (2024) reviewed medical and psychological databases from 2019 through 2020 to uncover research on family-centered interventions aimed to improve care of children with chronic illnesses (target was children 12 and younger in the sample) and their goal was to discover studies with ten or more participants (participants in studies ranged from 10 to 30 participants to over 300 participants). Family-centered care interventions were aimed at proving care that involved,

> …planning, delivery and evaluation of healthcare that was grounded in mutually beneficial partnerships among healthcare providers, patients, and families. We considered an intervention to be family-centered if: the main objective of the intervention was to improve healthcare experiences (including timely access to care or treatment, coordination of care, communication with providers and emotional support) for the population; and both (i) healthcare providers and/or administrators and (ii) primary caregivers of children were actively engaged in the development or research of the intervention (e.g., in the study of implementation of the intervention). (Chow et al., p. 4)

They found 63 studies with 61 interventions. Interventions most frequently focused on improving involvement of families in care and improving communication, while some targeted access. All studies need to include activities that would improve the family's healthcare experience. Most of the interventions addressed the family or parents and children with illnesses, although one intervention focused on siblings and 20 targeted care providers.

Chow et al. (2024) evaluated the interventions based on how many aspects of family-centered care were included. Care-coordination was often addressed by ensuring that the child had a range of services, delivered by a team with different types of expertise (a multidisciplinary team) where care was provided in the child's medical home or at one setting to offer a single point of care provision. Interventions also encouraged group meetings with the family to make decisions about care and share information about the child's progress. Other interventions included online platforms to share information (to encourage communication among the team and families) and engage practitioners and videos to educate parents and children (often about rehabilitation practices). One intervention redesigned a clinic's booking system, making appointments easier to access. Another study intervention educated parents so that they would be able to discuss their ideas about targets for treatment for their child.

When discussing their findings, Chow et al. (2024) mentioned that parent satisfaction with virtual platforms varied, and more research will be needed to optimize this method for improving communication and delivering information in a family-friendly way. Families with low digital literacy may need an intervention to train them about technology and those without computer access may need to be provided with computers or iPads to use at home, to make it easy for them to access information and communicate using technology. In terms of care coordination, team-based meetings with parents (and children where possible) remained a common method of improving communication and sharing interventions. In these meetings, families can build relationships with providers, making it easier to share information and ask questions, as well as share challenges to implementing interventions. Sharing challenges may become easier, once the family has built a relationship with providers. Importantly, Chow et al. (2024) recommended involving families in the design of interventions, and this could occur through working with an advisory group of parents and children with chronic illnesses to help design and monitor implementation of the interventions.

Family empowerment would build upon teaching communication, problem-solving, and how to care for the child's illness to improve self-efficacy for the child and family to manage the disease, which in turn, has the potential to improve quality of life. Mardhiyah et al. (2022) reviewed family empowerment studies in three databases (from 2013 to 2022), including PubMed CINAHL, and Proquest, to examine outcomes of studies with interventions for family empowerment. They found nine studies, four were quasi-experimental, four were experimental, and one was a pilot study. Most interventions addressed increasing family knowledge (child and parent knowledge) about care for the disease, increasing self-efficacy for disease management, and improving confidence for disease care, often through participatory training. Outcomes included positive change in feelings of self-efficacy and quality of child and family life. Mardhiyah et al. (2022) proposed that increases in family empowerment could reduce the length of stay in medical facilities and medical appointments. However, they searched a limited number of databases, and it was noteworthy that they did not search psychological databases. Nonetheless their findings to seem consistent with the notion of strengthening family resilience to improve family life and coping with a child's illness (Walsh, 2013).

Ren et al.'s (2024) study supports and extends the discussion by Mardhiyah et al. (2022), although their focus was on family resilience, rooted in Walsh's (2013) ideas. Ren et al. (2024) conducted a Delphic poll, with three rounds of feedback, with 14 experts in family care and resilience to determine critical concepts for improving family resilience for coping when a child has a chronic illness. Their findings overlap ideas presented by Chow et al. (2024). They mentioned that resilience of the family could be increased by strengthening family beliefs, adjusting family organization patterns to cope with the child's illness, and improving family communication. Specifically, health and mental health providers can foster family resilience by helping them use their internal and external resources to cope with the demands of or needs related to the child's illness. For instance, an internal strength might be the ability to problem-solve related to making family dinners appetizing for everyone, including the child with an illness, if their tastes change. An external resource might be a grandparent willing to babysit other children in the family, when parents need to attend medical appointments or be in the hospital with the child. Stressing cooperative problem-solving—how the family can work as a team and network with providers at the child's medical home to improve care of the illness, is another factor that will improve family resilience. Communication styles that are practiced with family members, which enhance listening and empathy skills may also improve family functioning and coping. Part of improving listening skills should be training in listening to the child's needs, perceptions, and beliefs—as they may want to communicate that they want more chances to be children and have fun. In fact, they may have differing perceptions of their lives compared to what parents believe their lives to be like, having more positive perceptions of their quality of life than their parents do (Hall et al., 2019).

Conclusion

The information in this chapter presents a review of the impact and nature of chronic illnesses and developmental disabilities for children and their families. It is our hope that this chapter orients readers to the nature of the conditions, so that readers may begin to reflect on ways to assist young children in schools as well as provide a glimpse of the importance of interventions to help children in their communities. Involving teachers and school nurses and considering and RTI and UDL approach ensures a systematic approach based on child needs and abilities as well as their needs in different spaces. Family-centered care and family-based interventions are ways to ensure that families can adhere to medical recommendations and make the interventions work to ensure success for the young child. We think that both an RTI/UDL and family-centered approach will improve the impact of community interventions for young children. The success of inclusion and interventions to foster development is enhanced by teamwork, that is, involving healthcare professionals, family, school, and community professionals in planning, executing, and assessing the impact of interventions to foster inclusion and child academic social, and emotional development. Interactions and being involved in play with peers in real-world settings will improve the social and emotional development of children (e.g., Nijhof et al., 2018; Saran et al., 2023). RTI and UDL, within a framework of family-centered care and teamwork to plan interventions, has the potential to improve inclusion and facilitate the academic success of young children.

References

AlRawi, J. M., & AlKahtani, M. A. (2021). Universal design for learning for educating students with intellectual disabilities: A systematic review. *International Journal of Developmental Disabilities, 68*(6), 800–808. https://doi.org/10.1080/20473869.2021.1900505

American Institutes for Research. (2025). *Center on multi-tiered systems of supports: Progress monitoring.* Retrieved from: https://mtss4success.org/essential-components/progress-monitoring

Anastasiou, D., Wiley, A. L., & Kaufman, J. M. (2024). A critical analysis of theoretical underpinnings of Universal Design for Learning. *Exceptionality.* https://doi.org/10.1080/09362835.2024.2426801

Arias-Gundin, O., & Llamazares, A. G. (2021). Efficacy of the RTI Model in the treatment of reading learning disabilities. *Education Sciences, 11*, 209. https://doi.org/10.3390/educsci11050209

Armendariz, G., & Jung, A. (2016). Response to Intervention vs. the Severe Discrepancy Model: Identification of students with specific learning disabilities. *The Journal of Special Education Apprenticeship, 5*(1), 1–18. https://doi.org/10.58729/2167-3454.1048

Aspiranti, K., Hilton-Prillhart, A., Bebech, A., & Dula, M. E. (2019). Response to Intervention (RTI) and the impact on school psychologist roles: Perceptions and acceptance of systems change. *Contemporary School Psychology, 23*, 327–337. https://doi.org/10.1007/s40688-019-00243-2

Barnett, T., Tollit, M., Ratnapalan, S., Sawyer, S. M., & Kelaher, M. (2023). Education support services for improving school engagement and academic performance of children and adolescents with a chronic health condition. *The Cochrane Database of Systematic Reviews, 2*(2), CD011538. https://doi.org/10.1002/14651858.CD011538.pub2

Barrio Cortes, J., Suárez Fernández, C., Bandeira de Oliveira, M., Muñoz Lagos, C., Beca Martínez, M. T., Lozano Hernández, C., & Del Cura González, I. (2020). Enfermedades crónicas en población pediátrica: comorbilidades y uso de servicios en atención primaria [Chronic diseases in the paediatric population: Comorbidities and use of primary care services]. *Anales de pediatria, 93*(3), 183–193. https://doi.org/10.1016/j.anpedi.2019.12.019

Berkeley, S., Scanlon, D., Bailey, T. R., Sutton, J. C., & Sacco, D. M. (2020). A snapshot of RTI implementation a decade later: New picture, same story. *Journal of Learning Disabilities, 53*(5), 332–342. https://doi.org/10.1177/0022219420915867

Blackwell, C. K., Elliott, A. J., Ganiban, J., Herbstman, J., Hunt, K., Forrest, C. B., Camargo, C. A., Jr., & Program Collaborators for Environmental Influences on Child Health Outcomes. (2019). General health and life satisfaction in children with chronic illness. *Pediatrics, 143*(6), e20182988. https://doi.org/10.1542/peds.2018-2988

Bortfeld, H., & Bunge, S. A. (2024). *Fundamentals of developmental cognitive neuroscience.* Cambridge University Press.

Chow, A. J., et al. (2024). Family-centred care interventions for children with chronic conditions: A scoping review. *Health Expectations: An International Journal of Public Participation in Health Care and Health Policy, 27*(1), e13897. https://doi.org/10.1111/hex.13897

Delamater, A. M., Guzman, A., & Aparicio, K. (2017). Mental health issues in children and adolescents with chronic illness. *International Journal of Human Rights in Healthcare, 10*(3), 163–173.

Demetriou, A., Spanoudis, G., & Papadopoulos, T. C. (2024). The typical and atypical developing mind: A common model. *Development and Psychopathology*, 1–13. https://doi.org/10.1017/S0954579424000944

Edyburn, D. L. (2010). Would you recognize universal Design for Learning if you saw it? Ten propositions for new directions for the second decade of UDL. *Learning Disability Quarterly, 33*, 33–41. https://doi.org/10.1177/073194871003300103

Fornauf, B. S., & Erickson, J. D. (2020). Toward an inclusive pedagogy through Universal Design for Learning in higher education: A review of the literature. *Journal of Postsecondary Education and Disability, 33*(2), 183–199.

Hall, C. A., Donza, C., McGinn, S., Rimmer, A., Skomial, S., Todd, E., & Vaccaro, F. (2019). Health-related quality of life in children with chronic illness compared to parents: A systematic review. *Pediatric Physical Therapy, 31*(4), 315–322. https://doi.org/10.1097/PEP.0000000000000638

Hall, T. E., Meyer, A., & Rose, D. H. (2012). *Universal design for learning in the classroom: Practical Applications.* The Guilford Press.

Hallahan, D. P., Pullen, P. C., & Kaufman, J. M. (2024). *Exceptional learners: Introduction to special education* (15th ed.). Pearson.

Hitchcock, C., Meyer, A., Rose, D. H., & Jackson, R. (2005). Equal access, participation, and progressin the general education curriculum. In D. H. Rose, A. Meyer, & C. Hitchcock (Eds.), *The universally designed classroom: Accessible curriculum and digital technologies* (pp. 37–68). Harvard Education Press.

Hogan, J. A. (2024). Discrepancy Model to RTI: Gauging teacher preparedness for this shift in specific learning disability classification. *Journal of Research in Special Educational Needs.* https://doi-org.uc.idm.oclc.org/10.1111/1471-3802.12730

Hollingshead, A., Lowrey, K. A., & Howery, K. (2022). Universal Design for Learning: When policy changes before evidence. *Educational Policy, 36*, 1135–1161. https://doi.org/10.1177/0895904820955120

Hudson, T. M., & McKenzie, R. G. (2016). Evaluating the use of RTI to identify SLD: A survey of state policy, procedures, data collection, and administrator perceptions. *Contemporary School Psychology, 20*, 31–35.

IDEA. (2004). Individuals with Disabilities Education Improvement Act of 2004. 118 Stat. 2647.

Jaudes, P. K., & Mackey-Bilaver, L. (2008). Do chronic conditions increase young children's risk of being maltreated? *Child Abuse & Neglect, 32*(7), 671–681.

Joseph, L. M., Konrad, M., Cates, G., Vajcner, T., Eveleigh, E., & Fishley, K. M. (2011). A meta-analytic review of the cover-copy-compare and variations of this self-management procedure. *Psychology in the Schools, 49*(2), 122–136. https://doi.org/10.1002/pits.20622

Kennedy, M. J., Thomas, C. N., Meyer, J. P., Alves, K. D., & Lloyd, J. W. (2013). Using evidence-based multimedia to improve vocabulary performance of adolescents with LD: A UDL approach. *Learning Disability Quarterly, 37*(2), 71–86. https://doi.org/10.1177/0731948713507262. (Original work published 2014).

Mace, R. L. (1998). Universal design in housing. *Assistive Technology: The Official Journal of RESNA, 10*(1), 21–28. https://doi.org/10.1080/10400435.1998.10131957

Maki, K. E., Burns, M. K., & Sullivan, A. L. (2018). School psychologists' confidence in learning disability identification decisions. *Learning Disability Quarterly, 41*, 243–256. https://psycnet.apa.org/doi/10.1177/0731948718769251

Mardhiyah, A., Panduragan, S. L., & Mediani, H. S. (2022). Reducing psychological impacts on children with chronic disease via family empowerment: A scoping review. *Healthcare (Basel, Switzerland), 10*(10), 2034. https://doi.org/10.3390/healthcare10102034

Morgan, A. (2019). Contributing to global mental health: Can pediatric psychology extend our reach? *Clinical Practice in Pediatric Psychology, 7*(2), 157–169. https://doi.org/10.1037/cpp0000282

National Center for Response to Intervention. (2010). *Essential components of RTI: A closer look at Response to Intervention.* Retrieved from: https://files.eric.ed.gov/fulltext/ED526858.pdf

Newacheck, P. W., & Halfon, N. (1998). Prevalence and impact of disabling chronic conditions in childhood. *American Journal of Public Health, 88*(4), 610–617.

Newacheck, P. W., & Taylor, W. R. (1992). Childhood chronic illness: Prevalence, severity, and impact. *American Journal of Public Health, 82*(3), 364–371. https://doi.org/10.2105/ajph.82.3.364

Nijhof, S. L., Vinkers, C. H., van Geelen, S. M., Duijff, S. N., Achterberg, E. J. M., van der Net, J., Veltkamp, R. C., Grootenhuis, M. A., van de Putte, E. M., Hillegers, M. H. J., van der Brug, A. W., Wierenga, C. J., Benders, M. J. N. L., Engels, R. C. M. E., van der Ent, C. K., Vanderschuren, L. J. M. J., & Lesscher, H. M. B. (2018). Healthy play, better coping: The importance of play for the development of children in health and disease. *Neuroscience and Biobehavioral Reviews, 95*, 421–429. https://doi.org/10.1016/j.neubiorev.2018.09.024

Nilvius, C., Carlsson, R., Fälth, L., & Nordström, T. (2021). Tier 2 interventions within the RtI-model for developing students' word decoding—A systematic review and meta-analysis. *Cogent Education, 8*(1), 1994105.

Nur, A. B. S. S., Chua, J. Y. X., & Shorey, S. (2023). Effectiveness of community-based family-focused interventions on family functioning among families of children with chronic health conditions: A systematic review and meta-analysis. *Family Process, 62*, 1408–1422. https://doi.org/10.1111/famp.12930

Ok, M. W., Rao, K., Bryant, B. R., & McDougal, D. (2017). Universal Design for Learning in pre-k to grade 12 classrooms: A systematic review of research. *Exceptionality, 25*(2), 116–138. https://doi.org/10.1080/09362835.2016.1196450

Perrin, J. M., Bloom, S. R., & Gortmaker, S. L. (2007). The increase of childhood chronic conditions in the United States. *JAMA, 297*(24), 2755–2759.

Ren, L., Wang, Y., Jiang, H., Chen, M., Xia, L., & Dong, C. (2024). Development of a theory-based family resilience intervention program for parents of children with chronic diseases: A Delphi study. *Journal of Pediatric Nursing, 74*, 41–50. https://doi.org/10.1016/j.pedn.2023.11.020

Rose, D. H., & Meyer, A. (2002). *Teaching every student in the digital age: Universal design for learning*. Association for Supervision and Curriculum Development.

Saran, A., Hunt, X., White, H., & Kuper, H. (2023). Effectiveness of interventions for improving social inclusion outcomes for people with disabilities in low- and middle-income countries: A systematic review. *Campbell Systematic Reviews, 19*(1), e1316. https://doi.org/10.1002/cl2.1316

Skinner, C. H., McLaughlin, T. F., & Logan, P. (1997). Cover, copy, and compare: A self-managed academic intervention effective across skills, students, and settings. *Journal of Behavioral Education, 7*, 295–306. https://psycnet.apa.org/doi/10.1023/A:1022823522040

U.S. Department of Education. (2004). Individuals with disabilities education act. Public Law 108-446. https://www.congress.gov/bill/108th-congress/house-bill/1350/text

U.S. Department of Education Statistics. (2024). Students with disabilities. Retrieved from: https://nces.ed.gov/programs/coe/indicator/cgg/students-with-disabilities#suggested-citation

U.S. Department of Health and Human Services. (2023). Diagnosed developmental disabilities in children aged 3–17 years: United States, 2019–2021. Retrieved from: https://nces.ed.gov/programs/coe/pdf/2024/CGG_508c.pdf

Unal, N. U., Karal, M. A., & Tan, S. (2022). Developing accessible lesson plans with Universal Design for Learning (UDL). *International Journal of Disability, Development, and Education, 69*(4), 1442–1456. https://doi.org/10.1080/1034912X.2020.1812539

van der Lee, J. H., Mokkink, L. B., Grootenhuis, M. A., Heymans, H. S., & Offringa, M. (2007). Definitions and measurement of chronic health conditions in childhood: A systematic review. *JAMA, 297*(24), 2741–2751. https://doi.org/10.1001/jama.297.24.2741

Walsh, F. (2013). Community-based practice applications of a family resilience framework. In D. Becvar (Ed.), *Handbook of family resilience* (pp. 65–82). Springer. https://doi.org/10.1007/978-1-4614-3917-2_5

Watkinson, M. D., Ehlenbach, M., Chung, P. J., Kelly, M., Werner, N., Jolliff, A., Katz, B., Marleau, H., Nacht, C. L., Warner, G., & Coller, R. J. (2023). Interventions in the home and community for medically complex children: A systematic review. *Pediatrics, 151*(5), e2022058352. https://doi.org/10.1542/peds.2022-058352

Zhang, L., Carter, R. A., Greene, J. A., & Bernacki, M. L. (2024). Unraveling challenges with the implementation of Universal Design for Learning: A systematic literature review. *Educational Psychology Review, 36*. https://doi.org/10.1007/s10648-024-09860-7

Chapter 2
Promoting Inclusion and Belonging in Religious Settings

Erik W. Carter

Abstract This chapter examines how religious congregations can move from inadvertent exclusion to faithful inclusion of children with developmental disabilities and their families. It proposes a ten-dimension framework of belonging—included, invited, welcomed, known, accepted, supported, heard, befriended, needed, and loved—and recommends congregational postures and practices in each area. Guided by universal design, the chapter urges proactive planning that anticipates diverse abilities, prioritizes flexible worship and learning, and centers family voices in decision-making. It highlights the mixed experiences of families, addresses attitudes and supports required for meaningful participation, and calls for intentional outreach and partnerships with disability organizations. Finally, the chapter identifiest research priorities focused on advancing a vision of faith communities where all children belong and flourish.

Keywords Religion · Spirituality · Faith · Developmental disabilities · Chronic illness

The embrace of a loving community can make a profound difference in the lives of children with disabilities and their families. Access to strong services, evidence-based practices, and high-quality programs matter immensely. But the experience of being known, needed, befriended, and beloved is at the heart of real flourishing for many families. Like anyone else, children with disabilities and their families want to be welcomed within communities in which they are seen as integral and invaluable members (Carter, 2021b).

Faith communities hold great potential as places of inclusion and belonging for these families. Although local congregations can vary widely in their beliefs, members, and ways of gathering, most share a deep commitment to building authentic community around shared values, rituals, and lives. The opportunities they offer

E. W. Carter (✉)
Baylor Center for Disability and Flourishing, Baylor University, Waco, TX, USA
e-mail: erik_carter@baylor.edu

L. Nabors and T. Stanton-Chapman (eds.), *Developmental Disabilities and Chronic Illness in Young Children*, Springer Series on Child and Family Studies,
https://doi.org/10.1007/978-3-032-08523-8_2

for people with and without disabilities to worship together, learn together, serve together, and grow together in their faith are often abundant. Yet, many faith communities still struggle to welcome and embrace this segment of their community (Carter, 2023; Stewart-Ginsburg et al., 2024). Indeed, the faith stories of children with disabilities and their families intermingle themes of both exclusion and embrace (Ault et al., 2013; Carter et al., 2025a). In the absence of guidance and support, most local congregations are prone to gather in ways that overlook or omit these essential members.

This chapter focuses on the practices and postures of congregations that can help children with disabilities and their families flourish in their faith. Although the religious lives of these families are rarely discussed in professional circles, faith can be an especially impactful dimensions of many family's lives (Carter, 2019; Lakhani et al., 2025). I review recent research on its importance, their religious involvement, and common barriers to congregational inclusion. Next, I introduce a practical framework for fostering belonging within faith communities and outline steps congregations can take to move in this direction. I conclude by highlighting several ways in which service systems and faith-based organizations can partner to support families in this area of their lives.

Spiritual Lives of Children and Their Families

Faith holds prominence in the lives of many children and families across the United States and around the world (Woodberry et al., 2025). The same is true for children and families who experience disability. Scores of studies highlight the prominent place religion and/or spirituality hold within these highly diverse families (see reviews by Carter, 2021b; Parchomiuk & Ćwirynkałob, 2025).

Importance and Impact

Although every family has a unique story in this space, several patterns emerge within research addressing the spiritual lives of children with disabilities and their families. First, faith has great importance to many of these families. A substantial proportion of parents of children with disabilities share that their faith matters, that it impacts their everyday decisions, and that prayer and other spiritual practices are a regular part of their lives (e.g., Boehm & Carter, 2019a; Holle et al., 2024). Second, faith can be a significant source of strength and resilience. Parents often express how their religious beliefs and practices provide meaning and direction, promote coping in the midst of everyday stressors, sustain them through life's challenges, and shape their interpretations of disability (Carter, 2019). Third, parents often share how their involvement in a faith community connects them with an array of much-needed practical, emotional, spiritual, and personal supports (Carter et al., 2016b). This might include a word of encouragement, an evening of respite, care through counseling, the gift of financial assistance, prayer amidst a medical issue, or the ongoing presence of a faithful friend. Finally, faith can contribute substantially to overall well-being. Studies show that individual and family quality of life can each be enhanced by one's spirituality and religious involvement (e.g., Carter, 2024; Boehm & Carter, 2019b; Poston & Turnbull, 2004).

At the same time, the faith stories of families navigating disability can also be challenging or crushing (e.g., Carter et al., 2025a; Salkas et al., 2016). Some parents struggle to reconcile their religious beliefs with the unanticipated realities of raising a child with developmental disabilities. They may blame God for a particular diagnosis, view certain conditions as form of punishment, question God's providence, or come to doubt God's existence. Other parents have felt bludgeoned by the errant beliefs of others. They may be told—and come to believe—that disability is the result of their sin, a lack of faith, or cosmic retribution; that their child with disabilities has less value and worth; or that their child is incapable of real faith. In such cases, religious beliefs can feel more hurtful than healing.

Involvement

The importance of faith often—though not always—leads toward involvement in a faith community. Many children with developmental disabilities and their families participate actively in the life of their church, mosque, synagogue, or other local religious congregation. Indeed, a growing number of state, regional, and national studies in the United States all point to high levels of involvement in worship services, religious education, rites of passage, and social events (e.g., Ault et al., 2013; Carter et al., 2016b; Koonan et al., 2020). For example, Whitehead (2018) found that three quarters of children with intellectual disability and two thirds of autistic children attended religious services at least annually. Likewise, Boehm and Carter (2019a) reported that most parents of children with developmental disabilities regularly attended worship services and participated in one or more other congregational activities. Qualitative studies further illustrate the myriad ways these parents are attending and serving within their faith community, as their children participate in religious education, summer camps, social events, and other activities (Carter et al., 2025b). Such active involvement may be especially salient within culturally and linguistically diverse families (e.g., Holle et al., 2024; Pearson et al., 2024).

Barriers

Although many families of children with disabilities are involved in a local congregation, their participation tends to be much more limited, more bounded, and more precarious than that of families whose children do not have disabilities. Indeed, some of these same studies highlight significant gaps between the participation of children with and without disabilities (Lee et al., 2008; Whitehead, 2018). Other studies point to the wide differences between the *desired* and *actual* involvement of children with disabilities and their families (Carter et al., 2016a; Howell & Pierson, 2010). For example, involvement tends to be less frequent for children with extensive support needs, behavioral challenges, communication needs, and complex medical issues.

A constellation of barriers can converge to hinder the meaningful participation of children with disabilities and their families in the congregation of their choice. Interviews involving parents of children with developmental disabilities highlight how barriers of awareness, architecture, attitude, and access can prevent families from engaging in congregational life in the ways and depth they would like (e.g., McMahon-Panther & Bornman, 2021; Pearson et al., 2024; Richardson & Stoneman, 2015). For example, in their interviews with 27 parents of children with developmental disabilities, Carter et al. (2025a) heard examples of 22 different barriers falling within nine primary areas: the commitments of leaders, the attitudes of fellow members, the prevailing expectations for participation, the availability of support, the capacity of volunteers, the accessibility of spaces, the ways information is communicated, the support needs of their children, and their own perspectives as parents. Within worship services, additional barriers can include the complexity of information, sensory issues, social expectations, theological beliefs, and more (Carter et al., 2024; Stewart-Ginsburg et al., 2024).

Moving from Barriers to Belonging

Faith communities committed to the meaningful inclusion of children with developmental disabilities and their families must be intentional in their efforts to foster inclusion and belonging. Inclusion is often thought of as being part of the programs and places that everyone else participates in. Belonging, however, is having the felt assurance that you matter within a community that matters to you. It entails a deeper level of connection that extends beyond merely sharing space or holding some affiliation in common. Instead, belonging is grounded in reciprocal relationships and mutual care. Although belonging is also an important pursuit in schools, neighborhoods, and community programs, it has special salience within faith communities (Carter, 2022a; Huggins & Copeland, 2023). Indeed, many religious communities recognize a theological call toward believing and belonging (Gaventa, 2021; Swinton, 2012).

In this section, I introduce a practical framework for fostering belonging in religious congregations that emerges from nearly two decades of research in this area (Carter, 2016, 2021a). Specifically, belonging is experienced when children with disabilities and their families are *included, invited, welcomed, known, accepted, supported, heard, befriended, needed,* and *loved* (Carter, 2021a; see Fig. 2.1). Each of the following sections highlights congregational practices and postures that can help weave children with disabilities and their families more fully into their faith community. Figure 2.2 displays a tool congregations can use to reflect on each of these ten dimensions of belonging.

Included The foundation for belonging is time spent together in the company of others. Such regular encounters—whether within the walls of the congregation or elsewhere in the wider community—create the context where meaningful relationships can grow. Children with disabilities and their families should participate in the same breadth of programs, places, events, and activities as anyone else. Different, separated, or segregated models of ministry for families impacted by disability ultimately limit the opportunities people have to meet and get to know one another. Congregations must be intentional about removing barriers that prevent the full participation of children with disabilities and their families. Especially important are barriers of awareness and attitude, invitation and imagination, commitment and culture, and theology and tradition.

Invited When children with disabilities and their families are absent from worship services, religious education, and social gatherings, the right remedy is intentional invitation. Some families may hesitate to engage in a faith community because of past wounds, fear of exclusion, or uncertainty about how they will be received. In response, congregations should reach out with warmth and care—extending genuine invitations to those who may be waiting to be asked.

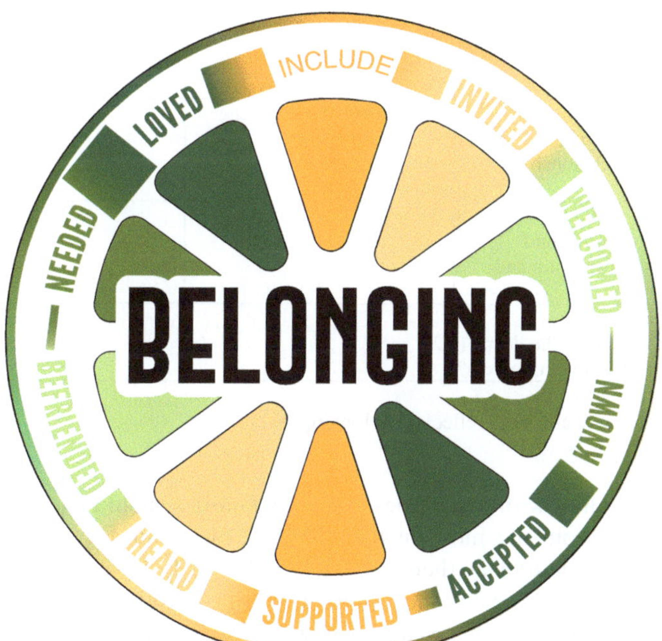

Fig. 2.1 Framework for fostering belonging in faith communities

Dimensions of Belonging	What are we doing **really well** right now?	How do we **know**?	What could we be doing **better** or **differently**?	What should we begin **doing next**?
Included Are children with disabilities involved in the experiences and events that are important to and for them?				
Invited Is their presence actively sought out by peers and others in their faith community?				
Welcomed Are they experiencing a warm and enthusiastic welcome whenever they arrive?				
Known Are they known personally and for the strengths and gifts they possess?				
Accepted Are they received graciously and unconditionally?				
Supported Are they receiving any assistance needed to participate fully and meaningfully?				
Heard Are their preferences and perspectives being sought on issues that matter?				
Befriended Are they developing and deepening their relationships with peers?				
Needed Are their talents, gifts, and contributions drawn upon and celebrated?				
Loved Are they experiencing the deep and unconditional love of others?				

Fig. 2.2 Congregational tool to reflect on belonging

Welcomed Children with disabilities and their families should encounter genuine warmth and joy from the moment they arrive. More than a mere greeting, true welcome conveys delight at their presence and signals they belong. Volunteers and leaders who have had limited experience with disability may need guidance or training on how to offer this welcome in ways that are both respectful and meaningful. Congregations should be intentional about shaping a culture of hospitality that not only accommodates—but actually celebrates—the arrival of every child and family.

Known Children with developmental disabilities are often seen through a limited lens—defined primarily by their challenges or perceived deficits (Patka & McDonald, 2015). A posture of belonging invites a broader, more affirming view: one that recognizes each child's strengths, gifts, interests, virtues, and more. When congregations take the time to know children with disabilities and their families in this way, the potential contributions they bring to the life of the community become much more evident. Congregations should intentionally seek out and celebrate the gifts and strengths each child has to offer.

Accepted Attitudes toward individuals with disabilities have long been mixed—even within communities of faith (Wang et al., 2021). Although congregations are called to be places where every child is fully embraced as valued and indispensable, children with disabilities and their families are sometimes still viewed through the lens of burden or limitation. The way a congregation speaks about disability—through preaching, teaching, and everyday conversations—can spread or stifle acceptance. When leaders model genuine welcome, invest in relationships, and speak with dignity and respect, they help create a culture where children with disabilities are seen as gifts. Congregations should promote awareness and understanding that leads to greater acceptance.

Supported Children with developmental disabilities and their families often need additional support to participate fully in the life of their congregation. Such support can take a variety of forms (see Fig. 2.3), but it should always emerge from ongoing conversations with families about what matters most to them. For example, leaders can adopt a posture of flexibility by adjusting how information is communicated, how children engage in activities, how assistance is offered, and how expectations are adapted to honor each child's unique needs. Likewise, support to families should focus on needs that are evident throughout the week and beyond the walls of the congregation (Carter, 2019). Congregations should be generous, imaginative, and proactive in their support of every child and family.

Heard The voices of children with disabilities and their families should always be valued within congregational decision-making. Too often, their needs are considered only after programs, policies, and spaces have already been designed, requiring retroactive adjustments that signal they were never part of the original vision. Proactive congregations recognize the value of listening closely to the experiences, insights, and priorities of families. When leaders take time to ask, listen, and respond, they affirm that every family's lived experiences and unique perspectives matter. Congregations should cultivate a culture in which members with disabilities are regularly and meaningfully heard.

Befriended The friendships formed by children with disabilities and their families are at the heart of belonging. Such relationships can bring great joy, meaning,

For Children with Disabilities

- Support plans for religious education, worship services, and other involvement
- Modified or alternative activities or curriculum
- A buddy system
- Sensory tools (e.g., headphones, fidgets) or spaces
- Visual schedules or timers
- Training for volunteers on supporting children with disabilities

For Parents, Siblings, and Other Family Members

- Meeting with caregivers about their needs and desired involvement
- Respite care
- Spiritual counseling
- Support group for caregivers
- Support and encouragement for siblings
- Childcare at congregational events
- Financial support
- Help connecting to community resources

Fig. 2.3 Example congregational supports for children with disabilities and families

companionship, and support. When children with disabilities are rarely included or poorly supported, the opportunities they have to meet and make friends becomes especially limited. Likewise, when parents cannot participate regularly in congregational programs because they must attend to their child, a sense of isolation often emerges. Active efforts are needed to support shared activities in which everyone can meet and spend time with others in their community who share their interests and backgrounds. Likewise, intentional connections can be forged through buddy programs, small groups, and fellowship activities aimed toward these children and their families. Congregations should prioritize the fostering of lasting relationships among all members, especially those impacted by disability.

Needed As congregation members come to know each other well, they should identify ways for children with disabilities and their families to serve, lead, and share their gifts with others. Most ministry models are built upon the premise that families impacted by disability need to be served and cared for (Carter, 2022b). Yet these families also have untapped contributions to make that can enrich the entire faith community. Examples include helping with aspects of a worship service, serving on a hospitality team, assisting on a service project, and reaching out to others in need. Congregations should seek out ways for children with disabilities and their families to serve and support others.

Loved The long-haul, unconditional love of a faith community can shape the lives of children with disabilities and their families in profound ways. Although service systems can offer invaluable resources, they are not built for love. Families also need to be surrounded by people who choose to remain in their lives—who see them, delight in them, and journey alongside them through joy and hardship alike. Congregations should be communities in which love abounds in word and deed.

Pathways to Inclusion and Belonging

The pursuit of greater inclusion and belonging for families of children with disabilities will require intentional and ongoing investment within most faith communities. Congregations exist across a broad continuum of commitment, programming, support, and resources related to the area of disability and religious ministry (Stewart-Ginsburg et al., 2024). As a result, their journeys and destinations will each look different as they try to respond faithfully to the clear call to welcome children and families residing in their midst. This section addresses six actions congregations can take to move forward.

Reflecting Together

More than 350,000 churches, synagogues, mosques, and other religious congregations exist in cities and counties throughout the United States (Association of Religion Data Archives, 2025). Each gathers in ways and places that are unique from all others, even when they affiliated with the same denomination or tradition. Indeed, local congregations vary widely in their sizes, spaces, histories, members, beliefs, and much more. As a result, there is no prescribed pathway or established set of practices that will resonate with every faith community. Instead, each community should invest in a thoughtful and collaborative process of regular reflection.

A variety of tools have been developed to help congregations attend to salient aspects of their spaces, supports, practices, programs, beliefs, and expectations (e.g., Carter, 2007; Christian Reformed Church in North America, 2021; LaRocque & Eigenbrood, 2005; Vander Plaats, 2016). Drawing upon existing tools can be especially helpful for congregations that have limited history or expertise with accessibility. In addition, some guiding questions to consider include:

- *What have been the experiences of children with disabilities and their families, both in the recent past and at present?*
- *Are our sanctuaries, classrooms, and buildings accessible and inviting?*
- *Do our worship and teaching practices prioritize certain bodies, minds, and ways of encountering the world?*
- *Are we extending support in meaningful and personalized ways?*
- *What explicit and unspoken expectations for behavior and participation may be hindering involvement?*
- *How familiar are we with who lives in our community and is already connected to our congregation?*
- *What are the prevailing attitudes and beliefs that we hold about disability and inclusion?*
- *How are people with disabilities actively involved in shaping and leading various aspects of congregational life, including worship, service, and leadership?*

- *How prepared and supported are our staff and volunteers to welcome and respond to the needs of children with disabilities and their families?*

Carter (2017) outlined four key principles to guide meaningful reflection. First, this process should be collaborative, drawing on the insights and experiences of a diverse group of participants. Second, individuals with disabilities and their families must be central contributors, ensuring their voices shape the conversation. Third, reflection should encompass a wide range of congregational practices and settings to provide a holistic understanding. Finally, such reflection is not a one-time activity; it should be approached as a continual and evolving process.

Preparing Proactively

Many congregational leaders express uncertainty about how to meaningfully welcome and include children with disabilities in the life of their faith communities. Historically, training opportunities in this area have been limited, and few theological institutions offer substantive engagement with issues of disability and ministry (Annandale & Carter, 2014; Ault et al., 2023). Similarly, lay leaders and volunteers often lack familiarity with how to support the participation of children with disabilities or complex medical needs in congregational programs. Preparing congregations to broaden their welcome requires a multifaceted approach that includes: (a) cultivating greater awareness throughout the congregation about disability and its implications for belonging, (b) articulating a compelling theological rationale for inclusion and accessibility, and (c) offering targeted training for leaders and volunteers. Awareness can be fostered through initiatives such as disability-focused worship services, sermons, small group studies, curriculum units, or special events. A strong theological foundation can motivate congregations toward more faithful and inclusive forms of gathering. Finally, training efforts should address principles of universal and responsive design, as well as best practices for inclusive ministry (Carter et al., 2024; Newman, 2021).

Inviting Widely

Religious congregations should be proactive about outreach toward children with disabilities and their families, just as they would anyone else. Nearly one in six children has a disability that impacts their learning, relationships, or participation (National Center for Education Statistics, 2024). Likewise, one in four households has at least one member who experiences disabilities (Altman & Blackwell, 2016). Congregational leaders should develop a deeper understanding of the demographics and needs within their local communities, as well as the most effective means for communicating about available programs and supports. Partnering with disability organizations and advocacy groups can serve as a valuable pathway for building relationships, increasing awareness, and strengthening community ties. Additionally, congregations should critically assess the language, imagery, and messaging used in their websites and outreach materials to ensure they reflect a welcoming posture and clearly convey inclusive opportunities for participation and support.

Planning Supports

Children with developmental disabilities should receive the individualized supports necessary to participate fully and meaningfully in all aspects of congregational life. Yet studies find that most families are never approached by congregation leaders to discuss their children's needs or explore what accommodations might be helpful (Ault et al., 2013, 2023). Too often, assumptions are made, or necessary supports are inadvertently neglected. One proactive strategy is to collaborate with families in creating a written support plan. Such a plan can outline the specific areas of congregational involvement that are important for the child—such as participating in Sunday school, attending vacation bible school, or attending fellowship events. It can also identify the types of supports that would foster successful participation, including having a peer buddy, using visual schedules, developing a communication system, applying adaptive technology, modifying instructional methods, or offering sensory-friendly spaces (see Fig. 2.3). Equally important are the child's and family's preferences about how supports are delivered—who provides them, when they are offered, and how best to honor the child's dignity. Thoughtful planning not only helps remove barriers, it also communicates that every member of the body is valued and expected to belong.

Changing Culture

Congregations that are truly committed to fostering belonging for children with disabilities and their families must be willing to reimagine how they gather and whom they center. Although offering adaptations or offering alternative options can address immediate barriers, such strategies often reflect a reactive stance—addressing needs only after exclusion has occurred. A more proactive approach is marked by anticipation rather than accommodation. This involves designing worship, learning, fellowship, and service opportunities from the outset with the assumption that children will arrive with a wide range of abilities, communication preferences, support needs, learning styles, and ways of engaging with the world and others. For example, when planning Sunday school, leaders might choose materials that incorporate visual supports, hands-on activities, and flexible pacing—not simply as an accommodation for a particular child, but as a standard practice for all children. In worship, offering prayer stations, visual liturgies, or movement-based responses are ways of creating meaningful entry points anyone in a church. This posture aligns with the principles of universal design, which reduce the need to retrofit ministries later by making inclusion foundational rather than supplemental. Ultimately, these shifts require more than programmatic changes—they involve cultivating a congregational culture in which diversity of embodiment and experience is expected, welcomed, and celebrated. Leaders must embed this perspective into every layer of congregational life, from strategic planning to volunteer training, so that inclusion is not the responsibility of a few individuals but part of the shared identity of the whole faith community.

Advocating Outward

As faith communities lean more into inclusion, many come to recognize how the presence and participation of children with disabilities and their families enrich the life of their congregation (Carter, 2022b). As they grow in their empathy and understanding, they also deepen their theological commitments to justice and access (Raffety, 2022). This journey often brings into sharper focus the broader social and structural barriers that impede the full flourishing of families in other areas of life. In response, congregations can extend their witness beyond their own communities by advocating for access and reform in areas like schooling, housing, employment, social services, and more. They may also partner with other congregations to advance disability justice across the wider community. In other words, they begin calling others to embody what their congregation is living out and discovering.

Future Research Directions

Research at the intersection of faith and disability is still an emerging field of study (see reviews by Carter, 2023; McMahon-Panther & Bornman, 2025). Although theological scholarship now seems to be surging, empirical research has remained far more limited. There is a pressing need for rigorous and interdisciplinary research that addresses the experiences of children with disabilities and their families, evaluates congregational practices, and identifies sustainable pathways toward deeper inclusion and belonging in faith communities. Several key areas of research stand out as especially urgent.

First, our understanding of the current practices and prevailing postures of local congregations in relation to disability is still limited. Although interviews with families suggest wide variability across faith communities, the field lacks systematic data on the actual supports, structures, and strategies in place—or absent—within these settings. Research should extend beyond self-reported surveys to include ethnographic fieldwork, direct observations in congregational settings, and mixed-method approaches that examine how inclusion (or exclusion) is enacted in real-time and over time.

Second, little is known about the mechanisms through which real and lasting change is initiated and sustained in congregational life. Despite growing awareness of inclusion as a theological and moral imperative, most congregations remain early in their journeys toward full accessibility and belonging. Research is needed to uncover the catalysts of change—such as the influence of leaders, the salience of training, the importance of theological reflection, and the role of community partnerships—and how these (and other) forces interact over time. This area of inquiry could benefit from drawing on implementation science, organizational change theories, and literature from adjacent fields such as inclusive education, integrated employment, and community inclusion. At the same time, researchers must also attend carefully to the unique values, resources, structures, and rhythms that shape religious communities.

Third, more imaginative and child-centered approaches to exploring the spiritual lives and faith formation of children with developmental disabilities are needed. Much of the current literature centers the perspectives of parents or ministry leaders, with limited direct engagement with children themselves. Given the diversity of communication styles and support needs evident among children with developmental disabilities, researchers must develop creative method for data collection to capture the voices, values, and spiritual expressions of children. Longitudinal studies are also needed to trace how their faith identities and personal practices develop over time.

Fourth, the field needs large-scale, nationally representative studies to understand broader patterns and benchmarks across faith communities. Most previous research is based on small, non-random, and often regionally bound convenience samples. National surveys involving parents, clergy, religious educators, and lay leaders could provide new insights into prevailing beliefs, perceived barriers, current practices, and unmet needs. Such studies could also identify differences by denomination, region, congregation size, or other contextual factors, helping to inform both policy and practice at broader scales.

Fifth, future studies should explore the diversity of families and faith traditions—both within the United States and globally. To date, research has emphasized Christian and Western contexts. Future studies must intentionally include the voices of families from racially, ethnically, and socioeconomically diverse backgrounds, as well as those affiliated with other religious traditions. Cross-cultural research could illuminate both commonalities and culturally specific approaches to disability, faith, and community belonging, offering a richer and more inclusive foundation for shared learning and coordinated advocacy.

Implications for Practice

Supporting the spiritual lives of children with developmental disabilities requires collaborative engagement across disability services, faith communities, and families. Each has a distinct yet complementary role to play in fostering inclusion and ensuring that all children have opportunities to belong, grow, and flourish within their preferred religious communities.

Disability service systems have a vital role in supporting the spiritual lives of individuals with developmental disabilities. Best practices in person-centered planning emphasize the importance of recognizing and honoring each person's beliefs, values, and spiritual commitments (Carter, 2024). Yet most professionals receive little training in navigating this dimension of support. Agencies should examine their policies on spirituality, integrate relevant content into staff training, and build partnerships with local faith communities.

Although many faith communities express a commitment to access and inclusion, the actual experiences of children with disabilities and their families suggest a more uneven landscape. To move from intention to impact, faith communities must address barriers related to architecture, accessibility, attitudes, and awareness. Practical steps might include offering disability inclusion workshops, creating accessible spaces and programs, inviting feedback from individuals and families, and reviewing policies around participation and leadership.

Third, parents have the most prominent role in supporting the spiritual lives of their children with developmental, yet they often wonder how to do this well (Carter et al., 2025a). Providing families with resources can equip them to nurture both spiritual growth and congregational connection. At the same time, caregivers also need spiritual support for themselves. Access to pastoral care, support groups, respite, or faith-based retreats can all enhance family well-being and resilience over the long term.

References

Altman, B. M., & Blackwell, D. L. (2016). Disability in U.S. households, 2000–2010: Findings from the National Health Interview Survey. *Family Relations, 63*(1), 20–38. https://doi.org/10.1111/fare.12044

Association of Religion Data Archives. (2025). *United States membership report:* 2020. https://www.thearda.com/

Ault, M. J., Collins, B. C., & Carter, E. W. (2013). Congregational participation and supports for children and adults with disabilities: Parent perceptions. *Intellectual and Developmental Disabilities, 51*(1), 48–61. https://doi.org/10.1177/0014402915598773

Ault, M. J., Slocum, V., Collins, B. C., Leahy, M. M., & Miller, V. P. (2023). Perceptions of faith leaders on the inclusion and participation of individuals with disabilities in their communities. *Journal of Disability & Religion, 27*(1), 138–159. https://doi.org/10.1080/23312521.2021.1932691

Boehm, T. L., & Carter, E. W. (2019a). Facets of faith: Spirituality, religiosity, and parents of individuals with intellectual disability. *Intellectual and Developmental Disabilities, 57*(6), 512–526. https://doi.org/10.1352/1934-9556-57.6.512

Boehm, T. L., & Carter, E. W. (2019b). Family quality of life and its correlates among parents of children and adults with intellectual disability. *American Journal on Intellectual and Developmental Disabilities, 124*(2), 99–115. https://doi.org/10.1352/1944-7558-124.2.99

Carter, E. W. (2007). Including people with disabilities in faith communities: A guide for service providers, families, and congregations. Brookes.

Carter, E. W. (2016). A place of belonging: Research at the intersection of faith and disability. *Review & Expositor, 113*(2), 167–180. https://doi.org/10.1177/0034637316637861

Carter, E. W. (2017). From barriers to belonging for people with disabilities: Promising pathways toward inclusive ministry. In A. J. Johnson, R. Nelson, & E. M. Lund (Eds.), *Religion, disability, and gender violence* (pp. 25–44). Springer. https://doi.org/10.1007/978-3-319-56901-7_3

Carter, E. W. (2019). Spirituality and the family unit. In B. Turns, J. Ramisch, & J. Whiting (Eds.), *Systematically treating autism: A guide for empowering families* (pp. 179–187). Routledge.

Carter, E. W. (2021a). Dimensions of belonging for individuals with intellectual and developmental disabilities. In J. L. Jones & K. L. Gallus (Eds.), *Belonging and resilience in individuals with intellectual and developmental disabilities: Community and family engagement* (pp. 13–34). Springer.

Carter, E. W. (2021b). Spirituality and supports for individuals with intellectual and developmental disabilities and their families. In L. M. Glidden, L. Abbeduto, L. L. McIntyre, & M. J. Tassé (Eds.), *APA handbook on intellectual and developmental disabilities* (pp. 419–442). American Psychological Association.

Carter, E. W. (2022a). A place of belonging: Including individuals with significant disabilities in faith communities. *Inclusive Practices, 1*(1), 6–12. https://doi.org/10.1177/2732474520977482

Carter, E. W. (2022b). The changing landscape of disability and ministry in the church. *Currents in Theology and Mission, 49*(3), 4–9. https://currentsjournal.org/index.php/currents/issue/view/69

Carter, E. W. (2023). Research on disability and congregational inclusion: What we know and where we might go. *Journal of Disability & Religion, 27*(2), 179–209. https://doi.org/10.1080/23312521.2022.2035297

Carter, E. W. (2024). Spirituality, disability, and quality of life. *Journal of Policy and Practice in Intellectual Disabilities, 21*(1), 1–5. https://doi.org/10.1111/jppi.12458

Carter, E. W., Biggs, E. E., & Boehm, T. L. (2016a). Being present versus having a presence: Dimensions of belonging for young people with disabilities and their families. *Christian Education Journal, 13*(1), 127–146. https://doi.org/10.1177/073989131601300109

Carter, E. W., Boehm, T. L., Annandale, N. H., & Taylor, C. (2016b). Supporting congregational inclusion for children and youth with disabilities and their families. *Exceptional Children, 82*(3), 372–389. https://doi.org/10.1177/0014402915598773

Carter, E. W., Tuttle, M., Spann, E., Ling, C., & Jones, T. B. (2024). Toward accessible worship: The experiences and insights of Christians with disabilities. *Journal of Disability & Religion, 28*(2), 189–219. https://doi.org/10.1080/23312521.2023.2197435

Carter, E. W., Maddox, K., Petit, M., Eshman, S. R., Escobar, M. V., Casper, G., & Le Shana, J. L. (2025a). Barriers to belonging: The church experiences of families impacted by disability. *Review of Religious Research.* https://doi.org/10.1177/0034673X251386820

Carter, E. W., Pettit, M., Maddox, K., Escobar, M. V., Eshman, S. R., Le Shana, J. L. & Casper, G. (2025b). Faithful belonging: Supporting families of children with disabilities in church. *Religious Education, 120*(5), 410–425. https://doi.org/10.1080/00344087.2025.2524976

Christian Reformed Church in North America. (2021). *Everybody belongs, serving together: Inclusive church ministry with people with disabilities.* Author.

Gaventa, W. (2021). Whose am I? Spiritual pathways into the heart of belonging. In J. L. Jones & K. L. Gallus (Eds.), *Belonging and resilience in individuals with intellectual and developmental disabilities: Community and family engagement* (pp. 79–96). Springer.

Holle, L., Longo, E., & Mogro-Wilson, C. (2024). A comparison in the importance of religious and spiritual beliefs among Latinx parents of children with disabilities. *Journal of Disability & Religion, 28*(2), 260–284. https://doi.org/10.1080/23312521.2023.2197438

Howell, E. J., & Pierson, M. R. (2010). Parents' perspectives on the participation of their children with autism in Sunday school. *Journal of Religion, Disability & Health, 14*(2), 153–166. https://doi.org/10.1080/15228961003622302

Huggins, D. W., & Copeland, S. R. (2023). Disability and belonging in an inclusive Christian faith community. *Inclusion, 11*(4), 271–285. https://doi.org/10.1352/2326-6988-11.4.271

Koonan, K., Reichman, N. E., Corman, H., & Jiménez, M. E. (2020). School and community involvement of adolescents with chronic health conditions. *Journal of Adolescent Health, 67*(4), 576–582. https://doi.org/10.1016/j.jadohealth.2020.02.028

Lakhani, A., Ali, T. S., Ashraf, D., & Roy, D. K. (2025). Exploring informal social support experiences and coping strategies in families raising a child with an intellectual disability. *The Family Journal, 33*(1), 150–171. https://doi.org/10.1177/10664807241283045

LaRocque, M., & Eigenbrood, R. (2005). Community access: A survey of congregational accessibility for people with disabilities. *Journal of Religion, Disability & Health, 9*(1), 55–66. https://doi.org/10.1300/J095v09n01_04

Lee, L., Harrington, R. A., Louie, B. B., & Newschaffer, C. J. (2008). Children with autism: Quality of life and parental concerns. *Journal of Autism and Developmental Disorders, 38*(6), 1147–1160. https://doi.org/10.1007/s10803-007-0491-0

McMahon-Panther, G., & Bornman, J. (2021). The perceptions of persons with disabilities, primary caregivers and church leaders regarding barriers and facilitators to participation in a Methodist congregation. *Journal of Disability & Religion, 27*(1), 39–85. https://doi.org/10.1080/23312521.2020.1859040

McMahon-Panther, G., & Bornman, J. (2025). Persons with disabilities in the Christian church: A scoping review on the impact of expressions of compassion and justice on their inclusion and participation. *Journal of Disability & Religion, 25*(1), 81–108. https://doi.org/10.1080/23312521.2024.2331461

National Center for Education Statistics. (2024). *Students with disabilities (Condition of Education).* U.S. Department of Education.

Newman, B. J. (2021). Worship as one: Varied abilities in the body of Christ. With Ministries.

Parchomiuk, M., & Ćwirynkałob, K. (2025). Religiosity and spirituality in the context of intellectual disability: A systematic research review. *International Journal of Developmental Disabilities.* Advance online publication. https://doi.org/10.1080/20473869.2025.2477620

Patka, M., & McDonald, K. A. (2015). Intellectual disability and faith communities: Perspectives of Catholic religious leaders. *Disability & Society, 30*(8), 1241–1258. https://doi.org/10.1080/09687599.2015.1090953

Pearson, J. M., Malone, K. M., Stewart-Ginsburg, J. H., Manns, L. D. C., Martin, D. M., & Palazzo, K. M. (2024). "We should all be welcome:" A discourse analysis of religious coping for black parents raising autistic children. *Journal of Disability & Religion, 28*(2), 235–259. https://doi.org/10.1080/23312521.2023.2178993

Poston, D. J., & Turnbull, A. P. (2004). Role of spirituality and religion in family quality of life for families of children with disabilities. *Education and Training in Developmental Disabilities, 39*(2), 95–108.

Raffery, E. (2022). *From inclusion to justice: Disability, ministry and congregational leadership.* Baylor University Press.

Richardson, E. W., & Stoneman, Z. (2015). The road to membership: The role of resilience in seeking and maintaining membership in a faith community for families of children with disabilities. *Journal of Disability & Religion, 19*(4), 312–339. https://doi.org/10.1080/23312521.2015.1093442

Salkas, K., Magaña, S., Marques, I., & Mirza, M. (2016). Spirituality in Latino families of children with autism spectrum disorder. *Journal of Family Social Work, 19*(1), 38–55. https://doi.org/10.1080/10522158.2015.1114060

Stewart-Ginsburg, J. H., Carter, E. W., Ault, M. J., Tanner, A., & Becker, C. (2024). A preliminary national survey of accessible features of churches in the United States. *Review of Religious Research, 66*(4), 631–648. https://doi.org/10.1177/0034673X241268649

Swinton, J. (2012). From inclusion to belonging: A practical theology of community, disability, and humanness. *Journal of Religion, Disability, & Health, 16*(2), 172–190. https://doi.org/10.1080/15228967.2012.676243

Vander Plaats, D. (2016). *There is no asterisk: Changing attitudes about disabilities through the 5 stages.* Elim Christian Services.

Wang, Z., Xu, X., Han, Q., Chen, Y., Jiang, J., & Ni, G. (2021). Factors associated with public attitudes towards persons with disabilities: A systematic review. *BMC Public Health, 21*, 1058. https://doi.org/10.1186/s12889-021-11139-3

Whitehead, A. (2018). Religion and disability: Variation in religious service attendance rates for children with chronic health conditions. *Journal for the Scientific Study of Religion, 57*(2), 377–395. https://doi.org/10.1111/jssr.12521

Woodberry, R. D., Johnson, K. A., Case, B., Bradshaw, M., VanderWeele, T. J., & Johnson, B. J. (2025). Religious centrality across 22 countries. *Scientific Reports, 15*, 15081. https://doi.org/10.1038/s41598-025-99183-6

Chapter 3
Making Inclusion Work in School Settings for Children with Developmental Disabilities and Chronic Illnesses

Tiara Saufley Brown and Sara Snyder

Abstract This chapter examines how schools can effectively support diverse learners through equitable, collaborative, and evidence-based practices. Grounded in the Department of Educational Foundations and Exceptionalities framework, the chapter outlines core principles of inclusive education, including universal design for learning, individualized supports, and culturally responsive pedagogy. It highlights the roles of interdisciplinary teams, family partnerships, and data-informed decision-making in creating accessible environments that address academic, behavioral, and health-related needs. Practical strategies focus on proactive classroom design, assistive technology, flexible assessment, and coordinated care for students with chronic conditions. The chapter also addresses policy contexts, implementation challenges, and sustainability through professional development and continuous improvement. By centering student strengths and belonging, it offers actionable guidance to transform school systems and practices to promote participation, learning, and well-being for all students.

Keywords Children with developmental disabilities · Children with illness · Classroom environment · Engagement · Pyramid Model · Universal Promotion · Multi-tiered System of Support

Making Inclusion Work in School Settings for Children with Developmental Disabilities and Chronic Illnesses

Teaching can be a highly stressful occupation. Many teachers struggle with self-doubt and self-criticism. This is often referred to as self-internalizing behaviors or self-efficacy (Barni et al., 2019). These internalized patterns of thought often stem

T. S. Brown (✉) · S. Snyder
Department of Educational Foundations and Exceptionalities, James Madison University, Harrisonburg, VA, USA
e-mail: brown3ts@jmu.edu

L. Nabors and T. Stanton-Chapman (eds.), *Developmental Disabilities and Chronic Illness in Young Children*, Springer Series on Child and Family Studies,
https://doi.org/10.1007/978-3-032-08523-8_3

from a lack of confidence and can lead to heightened stress levels, depression, and burnout (Jennings & Greenberg, 2009). When teachers have low self-efficacy and think negatively about their job performance, they have difficulty making decisions, have lower job satisfaction, and ultimately create a less positive environment for their students (Tschannen-Moran & Hoy, 2001). Teachers' inability to manage these internalized behaviors affects their well-being, reduces their pedagogical effectiveness, hinders their interactions with children, and negatively impacts overall student outcomes.

Impact of Teacher Well-Being and Self-Efficacy on Children

Teacher self-efficacy plays a crucial role in shaping the educational experience for children, as teachers with high self-efficacy tend to create more supportive and engaging learning environments (Tschannen-Moran & Hoy, 2001). Teachers' beliefs in their ability to effectively instruct directly affect students' confidence, engagement, and overall success in the classroom (Bandura, 1997). Figure 3.1 depicts four impacted areas of teacher well-being and self-efficacy on children: classroom environment, teacher-student relationships, academic achievement, and social and behavioral outcomes for children.

Classroom Environment and Engagement

Children, especially young students in preschool, rely on a classroom environment that is highly engaging for motivation. Typical early childhood classrooms are vibrantly colorful with engaging visuals. Additionally, early childhood teachers mimic this physical environment with a warm, welcoming, and positive demeanor. When teachers experience low levels of self-efficacy and higher levels of anxiety or depression, they are often unable to create the welcoming classroom environment they desire. Prior research shows that depressive symptoms can lead to reduced emotional availability and responsiveness from teachers (Agyapong et al., 2022). An engaging classroom environment stimulates children's curiosity and desire to learn. When children are actively involved in their learning process, they are often more motivated and focused (Wentzel & Brophy, 2013). Wang and Eccles (2012) found that a positive classroom climate, characterized by supportive teacher-student interactions and engaging learning activities, significantly predicts engagement in children. This is particularly important for children with developmental disabilities (DD) or chronic illnesses. A well-designed classroom that accommodates the needs of children with DD or chronic illness ensures that all students can participate in activities. This includes physical accessibility (e.g., wheelchair access), sensory-friendly spaces, and adaptive materials (Gupta et al., 2014).

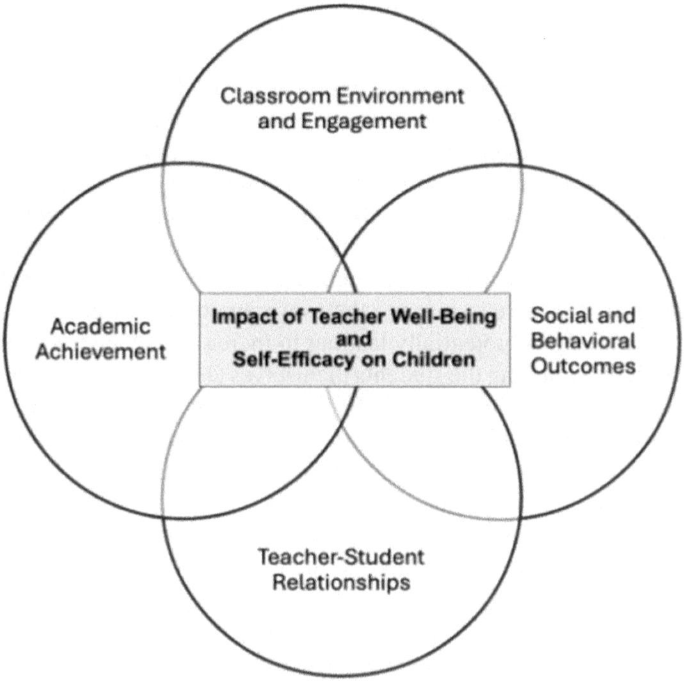

Fig. 3.1 Impact of teacher well-being and self-efficacy on children

Teacher-Student Relationships

Teacher-student interactions are crucial supports for children's development across domains including language, socioemotional, and academic success (Mashburn et al., 2008; Mortensen & Barnett, 2014). Ngyuen et al. (2020) found that preschoolers who had closer relationships with their teachers demonstrated enhanced improvements in all domains of school readiness. Teachers, who are managing depression or experience low levels of self-efficacy, may find it challenging to establish and sustain constructive relationships with their students. Teachers' social-emotional skills are fundamental in their capacity to create a supportive environment that promotes the social, emotional, and linguistic growth of young children.

The significance of relationships in early childhood environments is heightened in the context of inclusion. Carrington et al. (2016) found that early childhood educators recognized the advantages of inclusion for children with DD; however, they also expressed concerns regarding the challenges faced by teachers. This included heightened responsibilities, lack of adequate training, and time constraints. These findings suggest a need for implementing strategies aimed at enhancing teacher self-efficacy, thereby fostering positive relationships that will benefit young learners.

Social and Behavioral Outcomes

In addition to classroom relationships, Kwon et al. (2019) found that Early Head Start teachers with increased levels of depression reported more behavioral problems in their students. Their findings were consistent with previous research showing a link between depressive symptoms and teachers' inabilities to read cues from children or effectively respond to toddlers' needs, thus creating behavioral problems in the classroom (Hamre & Pianta, 2004). Similarly, Hamre and Pianta (2005) found that teachers' emotional states can influence students' emotional regulation and behavior. When teachers are less able to manage their own emotions, it can create a stressful environment for students, potentially leading to increased behavioral problems and emotional difficulties among the students themselves (Jennings & Greenberg, 2009).

Highly self-efficacious teachers are better at coping with classroom dynamics. They believe in their teaching abilities and create an enjoyable learning environment, which results in fewer behavioral problems for students (Klassen & Chiu, 2010). Additionally, effective and confident teachers are more adept at modeling conflict resolution, compassion, and cooperation. Children practice these behaviors when they see them, which can improve their social abilities. Teachers working with children who have DD and chronic illness must possess a strong sense of confidence in their capacity to apply tailored strategies that enhance positive social-emotional growth. Studies indicate that a teacher's self-efficacy in encouraging social skills plays a crucial role in achieving better results for children with DD, including heightened peer interactions and improved emotional regulation (Klassen & Chiu, 2010).

Academic Achievement

Finally, the academic achievement of young learners can be negatively impacted when their teachers are experiencing depression or are not confident in their teaching ability. Teachers exhibiting signs of depression frequently show a decrease in their teaching effectiveness, which is evident through lower energy and less effective instructional techniques (O'Connor & McCartney, 2007). This decline in teaching quality can lead to poorer student performance and a drop in academic motivation (McCormick et al., 2013). Additionally, students may experience heightened stress and anxiety regarding their academic achievement when their teachers are unable to provide the essential support and encouragement.

Research indicates that when children with DD receive customized instruction tailored to their specific learning requirements, they are more likely to attain significant advancements in academic achievement (Guralnick, 2011). Teachers who feel confident in their skills can provide a structured learning environment with proper accommodations and supports. Additionally, they are more likely to engage in effective collaboration with other educators, medical experts, and families to ensure students have access to appropriate learning experiences. This system of supports is critical to ensure young children with DD and chronic illness can develop foundational skills that set the stage for future academic success.

Coaching and Mentoring

The evidence of the impact on young learners, mentioned above, suggests a need for teachers to be confident in their instruction and positive in their interactions. Recognizing and addressing self-internalizing behaviors is essential for educators to fully fulfill their roles and responsibilities. Professional development (PD) and coaching, or mentoring, that emphasize emotional regulation and self-reflection, in addition to instructional strategies, can help teachers identify and manage their self-doubt (Sutton & Wheatley, 2003). By cultivating a supportive atmosphere and offering strategies for self-compassion and resilience, educators can enhance their self-efficacy and overall job performance.

Furthermore, data shows teacher turnover is increasing throughout the United States (Carver-Thomas & Darling-Hammond, 2019) which is linked to many factors including a lack of mentorship or coaching. Teachers often feel inadequate, unprepared, and strained with a heavy workload. Because quality education is intrinsically dependent on highly trained and dedicated teachers, enlisting coaching and mentoring for teachers is essential for young learners (Palacios, 2017). Ultimately, when early childhood educators confront these internalized challenges, they are better prepared to foster a nurturing and inclusive learning environment, thereby promoting their own professional growth and improving their students' developmental outcomes.

Laws and Professional Organizations for the Inclusion of Young Children

In addition to coaching and mentoring, teachers can rely on evidence-based practices from professional organizations to fully execute inclusion in their classrooms. Federal legislation advocates for the integration of young children with disabilities into natural environments, specifically the Individuals with Disabilities Education Improvement Act (IDEA) of 2004. This principle is also supported by prominent early childhood professional organizations, such as the Division for Early Childhood of the Council for Exceptional Children (DEC) and the National Association for the Education of Young Children (NAEYC). In their joint position statement on early childhood inclusion, DEC/NAEYC (2009) outline that high-quality inclusive programs and services are characterized by three essential features: access, participation, and supports. These features, when effectively implemented, enable educators to create environments where all children, regardless of ability, can thrive and engage meaningfully with their peers.

Moving Forward

Once a teacher has established a sense of self-efficacy, they are able to utilize evidence-based strategies to support the inclusion of young learners in many domains. The remainder of this chapter will discuss how teachers can adapt instruction for social/behavior and academic outcomes to include students with DD and chronic illness.

Supporting Social and Emotional Development for Young Children with Developmental Disabilities and Chronic Illnesses

Supporting social and emotional development in young children with DD and chronic illnesses is crucial for fostering their overall well-being and helping them navigate challenges in their daily lives. These children often face unique obstacles that can affect their ability to form meaningful relationships, express emotions, and adapt to social environments. By providing targeted support, individualized strategies, and inclusive environments, teachers can empower these children to build essential skills, enhancing their confidence, resilience, and emotional health.

Overview of the Pyramid Model

Challenging behaviors (CBs) may signal that a young child needs support to develop social-emotional skills (Price & Steed, 2016). CBs could occur with any child, including children with DD and chronic illnesses. The National Center for Pyramid Model Innovations (NCPMI, 2021) offers a tiered system of support for meeting the needs of all young children, depicted in Fig. 3.2. In the Pyramid Model, the base tier is 'Universal Promotion' and consists of practices meant to support all children through supportive environments and responsive relationships. The second tier is 'Secondary Prevention', which focuses on providing targeted support to young learners who need more assistance than what is provided to all children in the base tier. The third tier is 'Tertiary Intervention', which is designed to provide individualized and intensive help to young children who need social-emotional support beyond what is provided in Tiers 1 and 2. Classrooms and programs that utilize the Pyramid Model, or other

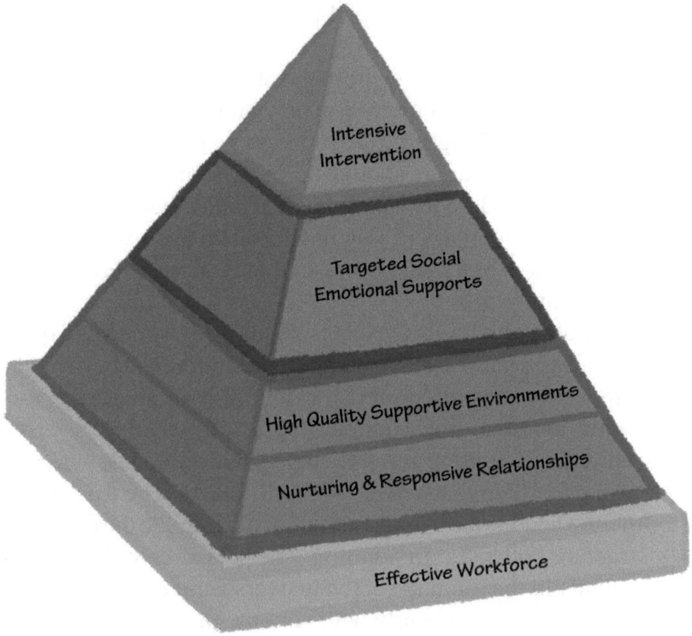

Fig. 3.2 The Pyramid Model for promoting social-emotional competence in infants and young children
Note: The NCPMI Pyramid Model graphic acquired from www.ncpmi.org

tiered intervention systems, promote inclusive environments where children at all stages of social and emotional development are supported (Rausch & Strain, 2021).

Tier 1: Universal Promotion

Universal promotion strategies are designed to support all children in inclusive settings, including children with disabilities and children at-risk for developing disabilities. This tier focuses on the teacher building nurturing relationships with young children. It includes implementing specific environmental arrangements and active supervision plans in all settings. Finally, this tier includes establishing, teaching, and re-teaching classroom expectations and routines that encourage children to engage in positive behaviors (Fox et al., 2021).

Responsive and nurturing relationships are essential for supporting social-emotional growth. This refers to relationships between teachers and young children, teachers and parents, and teachers and other adults. Responsive and nurturing relationships include positive time and attention, noticing and joining children's play, and giving directions that are brief and tell children what to do rather than focusing on what children should not do (Fox et al., 2021). Without responsive and nurturing relationships, the other strategies described in the Pyramid Model are not likely to be effective.

Additionally, it is critical to arrange the classroom environment to support young children's success. All learning areas need to be visible to supervising adults. There should be a variety of areas designed to accommodate groups of varying sizes. The boundaries of those learning areas should be clearly marked. However, teachers should take care to limit wide open spaces and arrange learning areas to promote safe traffic patterns in the classroom (NCPMI, 2021). For example, teachers will want to limit traffic through block play areas so that large structures are not knocked over onto other children.

Another Tier 1 strategy highlights teachers should clearly define expectations for learning areas and make plans to actively supervise children. They should establish and teach rules for how many children can safely play in an area as well as rules for safe play within the area. For example, the art center may be capped at 3–4 children so that children have ample room to engage with materials without disturbing other children also playing in that center (NCPMI, 2021). The teacher may need to implement a structure height rule in the block area to minimize the risk of injury when a large block structure collapses. In addition, teachers should develop supervision plans so that all adults in the room are actively overseeing children by scanning and moving throughout the room frequently while interacting with learners (Allen et al., 2019). This will help teachers ensure that learning areas are not overcrowded and that play within those areas are safe and appropriate.

Once expectations and rules are established, children will require explicit instruction throughout the year regarding how to follow rules and complete routines within and outside of the classroom. This instruction might focus on teaching children how to use a learning area, how to engage in classroom activities, how to transition from one activity to another, and expectations for mealtimes, etc. Instruction should include opportunities for student choice, and for the teacher to model expectations. Children should then have opportunities to practice the routine and receive feedback (Carter & Pool, 2012). Teachers should display visual supports showing children engaging in the expected behavior and refer to those supports often (Coleman et al., 2012).

Tier 2: Secondary Prevention

Most children will be successful with the universal supports described above. However, some will require additional behavioral and social-emotional supports to prosper in the inclusive setting. Tier 2 provides targeted social-emotional support for individual children or small groups, including those with developmental disabilities (DD) and chronic illnesses.

Before implementing Tier 2 strategies, the teacher should frequently examine their own behaviors, expectations, and biases. First, the teacher should seek to foster a nurturing and responsive relationship with the child if that relationship is not firmly established. Young children who engage in CBs are less likely to receive positive

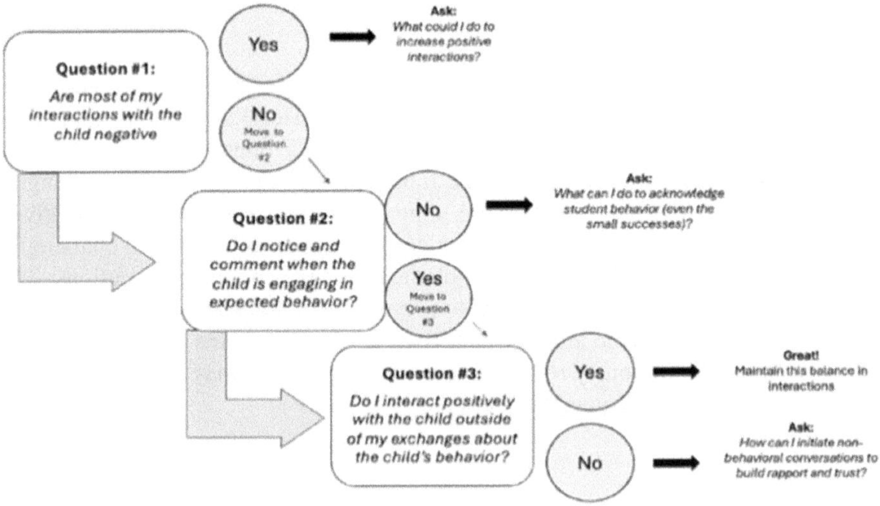

Fig. 3.3 Questions teachers should ask themselves when working with children who demonstrate challenging behavior

feedback from their teachers and more likely to have teacher interactions focused on challenging behavior than positive behavior (Hemmeter et al., 2012). Figure 3.3 depicts questions that teachers should continuously ask themselves when supporting a child who demonstrates challenging behavior.

Second, the teacher should assess their expectations for the child to ensure they are age-appropriate. This is especially important when supporting young children with DD and chronic illness. One way to do this is to compare the child's behavior to the behavior of another child in the setting who demonstrates *average* behavior and social-emotional skills. Then, the teacher should conduct observations and record data on the target child and comparison child. Are the children's behaviors and skills dramatically different? If not, maybe the teacher needs to reframe their expectations for the target child.

Third, the teacher should examine whether their expectations for the child are culturally appropriate. Children from culturally and linguistically diverse (CLD) backgrounds may present with behaviors that are considered appropriate at home, and in their community, but may not be acceptable at school. If this is the case, the child may require explicit instruction to learn what behaviors are appropriate for school. Another potential barrier may occur if child is struggling to convey all their needs in the school language, which may result in the child engaging in challenging behaviors in order to meet those needs (Barton & Banerjee, 2013). Barton and Banerjee (2013) note that culturally responsive teachers constantly examine their own beliefs, biases, and assumptions to meet the diverse needs of the children and families they serve.

Tier 3 Individualized Intervention

Tier 3 supports are specialized, individualized interventions for a child who needs more support than Tier 1 and 2. The child in need of Tier 3 supports demonstrates persistent challenging behavior that may be frequent or intense (Fox et al., 2021). Tier 3 supports focus on determining the function(s), or reason(s) why challenging behavior is occurring. This is a team-based process relying on input from caregivers and other service providers. Once the team determines the function(s) of challenging behavior, they can then develop and implement function-based interventions. This may include adapting the environment to prevent problem behavior from occurring or changing what people do after the challenging behavior occurs. Just like in Tier 2, teachers should continuously reflect on how their responses may impact the child's challenging behavior (Artman-Meeker et al., 2021).

Supporting Academic Instruction for Young Children with Developmental Disabilities and Chronic Illnesses

It is important that children with DD and chronic illnesses receive academic instruction in addition to social and behavioral supports. Early childhood teachers understand that rich learning experiences are imperative for young children. They must also remember that the child is a young learner first and they are not defined by their disabilities or medical conditions. Therefore, a teacher's primary goal should be the same as it is for any other student: play, learn, and develop relationships. All children deserve access to rich educational experiences and academic supports must be put into place to ensure all children have the opportunity to learn.

Overview of Multi-Tiered Systems of Support (MTSS) and Universal Design for Learning (UDL)

Similar to the Pyramid Model, Multi-Tiered Systems of Support (MTSS) is a system of targeted support for students who need assistance academically or behaviorally. MTSS can be used in early childhood settings to help identify at-risk students and help remedy potential developmental delays in young learners (Greenwood et al., 2019). MTSS is also separated into three tiers. In Tier 1, every student receives high-quality, core instruction in the general education classroom. In Tier 2, teachers provided targeted interventions for young learners who may require additional academic support. In Tier 3, teachers offer individualized and more intensive support to students with the most needs. Throughout these processes, teachers should monitor data closely to help guide decisions about student needs (Shepley & Grisham-Brown, 2019).

By using MTSS as a support system, teachers can then utilize Universal Design for Learning (UDL) to proactively help their students. According to Gauvreau et al. (2019), "UDL is a framework that supports the learning needs of all learners through intentional, proactive, and reflective instruction and interactions." The main goal of UDL is to encourage students take charge of their learning by giving them the power to make choices that help them reach their learning goals (Navaitienė & Stasiūnaitienė, 2021). Early educators can utilize this thoughtful design to adjust their planning, delivery, and assessment to promote inclusive practices.

UDL is a proactive, iterative, and intentional lesson design using guidelines and expert learning as the framework. Like MTSS and the Pyramid Model, UDL is also organized into three tiers. Teachers utilize Tier 1 for their proactive planning for all learners. In Tier 2 and 3, teachers can incorporate the specifics of UDL but differentiate instruction, assessment, and delivery for targeted supplemental interventions or individualized instruction (Gauvreau et al., 2019). Figure 3.4 shows how this process of incorporating UDL looks within the MTSS model (UDL and Multi-Tiered Systems of Supports (MTSS), n.d.)) Using MTSS and UDL simultaneously can help improve teaching for all young students (Thomas et al., 2023).

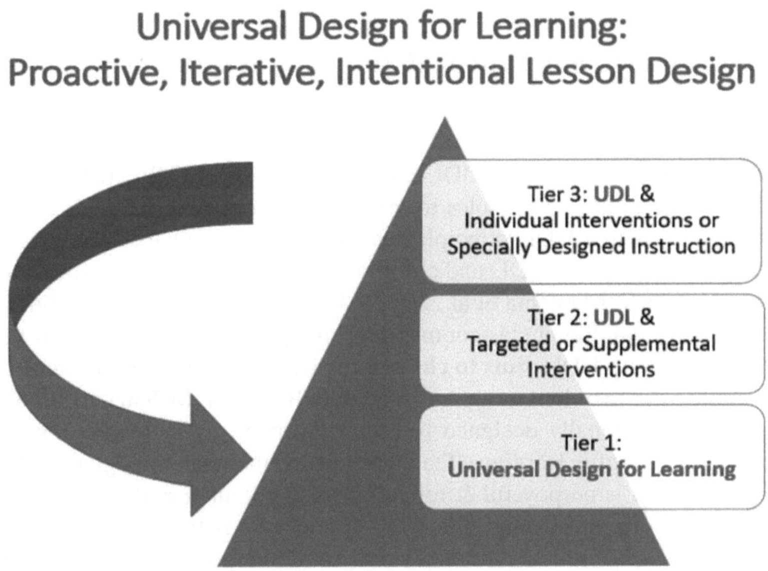

Fig. 3.4 Incorporating UDL within the MTSS Model
Note: This graphic shows how this process looks within the MTSS and UDL systems (acquired from https://www.sst6.org/UDLandMulti-TieredSystemsofSupportsMTSS.aspx)

Incorporating UDL into MTSS Framework in Our Scenario

The Center for Applied Special Technology (CAST) emphasizes how UDL can be utilized to improve the design of the environment. Teachers of young children can purposely plan their lessons to involve and engage every student in a meaningful way. When the environment and instruction are strategically planned, all students can take part in challenging and important learning. Using UDL principles, teachers can design a curriculum that is both easy to access and engaging. This approach encourages children with DD and chronic illnesses to actively take part in their learning.

Overall, UDL emphasizes that every child, regardless of disabilities or medical conditions, is first and foremost a young learner with inherent strengths and potential. Additionally, in order to ensure high-quality outcomes for all children in the early childhood classroom, teachers are expected to utilize both the Developmentally Appropriate Practices (DAPs) provided by NAEYC (2009a, 2009b), as well as the DEC Recommended Practices (DEC, 2014). Both NAEYC's DAP and DEC's Recommended Practices align with the use of UDL.

Principles of UDL and Practical Strategies for the Inclusion of Young Learners

After teachers understand how UDL can fit within the MTSS framework, they can utilize the three main principles to promote learner agency in their classroom. Research indicates that UDL principles can significantly enhance the educational experience for children with DD and chronic illnesses by improving accessibility in educational settings (Miedema et al., 2022). As more children with disabilities are included in early childhood classrooms, the principles of universal design become even more important. **UDL aims to change the design of the environment rather than to situate the problem as a perceived deficit within the learner.** When environments are intentionally designed to reduce barriers, every learner can engage in rigorous, meaningful learning. Teachers must remember the "goal of UDL is learner agency that is purposeful & reflective, resourceful & authentic, strategic & action-oriented". To ensure this, the UDL framework is built around three main components, seen in Fig. 3.5, often referred to as the guidelines, or three principles, of UDL: *multiple means of engagement, multiple means of representation, and multiple means of action and expression.*

Multiple Means of Engagement

The principle of multiple means of engagement focuses on strategies to engage student learning. Teachers must recognize that learners come from a variety of diverse

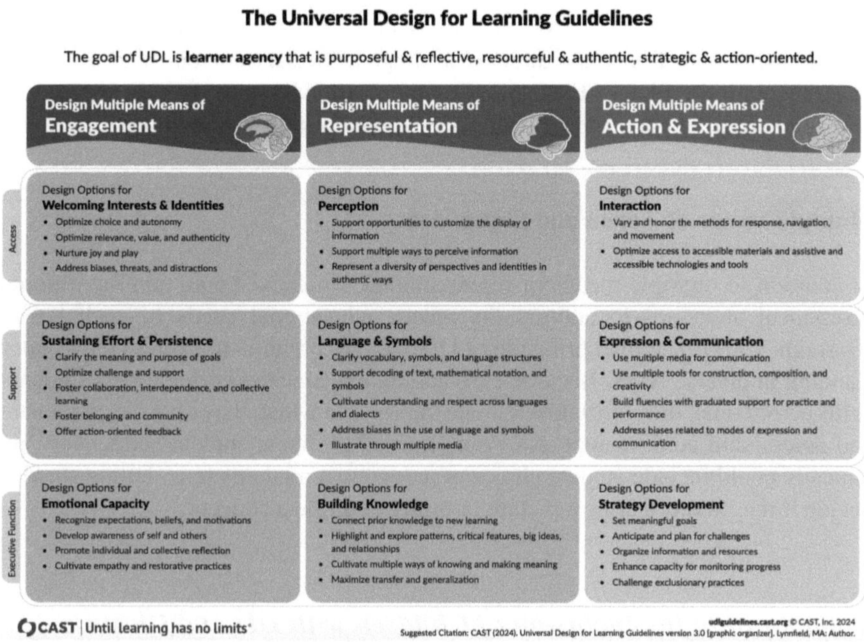

Fig. 3.5 The Universal Design for Learning guidelines
Note: The Center for Applied Special Technology (CAST) UDL guidelines acquired from udlguidelines.cast.org

backgrounds and abilities and must plan accordingly for engagement (Rappolt-Schlichtmann et al., 2013). Specifically, classroom arrangement is critical when fostering student learning through interactive lessons, movement, and play. In early childhood settings, teachers can offer choices in activities that cater to children's interests and preferences (e.g., offering different types of learning centers that cater to varying physical abilities and energy levels, giving students the option to choose between quieter, low-energy tasks or more active activities based on how they're feeling that day). They can also vary their teaching methods and materials, such as visual aids and tactile resources, to help children connect with the content in meaningful ways (Barrio & Hollingshead, 2017).

Multiple Means of Representation

Early childhood educators must acknowledge that children not only have different preferences, but they also comprehend information differently. The principle of multiple means of representation stresses that teachers should present information in a variety of ways to accommodate diverse learning needs (Gauvreau et al., 2019). This means that different students require varying formats and materials in order to access academic content. Teachers should present information in daily interactions and throughout various educational lessons in the classroom. One example could include using visual aids and audio recordings to present content (e.g., providing materials with the Picture Exchange Communication System (PECS) for students who are nonverbal or recording material for students with vision impairments).

Multiple Means of Action and Expression

In addition to multiple means of representation, teachers should employ different assessment strategies to address the unique educational needs of each learner (Darragh, 2007). The final principle of UDL allows children to express their understanding in diverse ways. Because early childhood educators often assess students' skills across time, they must differentiate the ways in which they observe, document, and assess skill achievement. An example used to assess students effectively and ethically could include student choice of assessment methods (e.g., letting students decide if they want to draw a picture or orally describe a concept).

Collaboration for Inclusion of Children with DD and Chronic Illness

Teachers may need support from other professionals in order to fully integrate UDL to instruct learners with DD and chronic illness. According to a recent study by Benson-Goldberg and Erickson (2024), early childhood educators reported spending an average of over 120 min per day providing academic instruction to students with extensive support and complex communication needs. This recent finding highlights the need for collaborations with related service providers.

There are a multitude of supports in public schools, but specifically for children with DD or chronic illness, a few key collaborative supports stand out. Interdisciplinary service delivery means that experts from different fields work together to help students succeed (Anderson, 2014). These team members are experts in their field and can utilize strategies from MTSS and UDL to work collaboratively for academic engagement.

First, early childhood educators must work with special education teachers. Special education teachers provide expert knowledge on how to adapt and modify general classroom instruction (Hunt et al., 2004). Teachers can work with special educators to effectively support students with DD and chronic illness to ensure students can access and participate in everyday lessons. Special educators also perform a variety of roles including writing and implementing IEPs, assessing children, ensuring legal compliance, assisting with accommodations and modifications, and preparing students for transition (Hunt et al., 2004).

For children with visual impairments (VI), early childhood educators can work with a Teacher of the Visually Impaired (TVI). TVIs are trained and certified to teach students with blindness or low vision (Fast, 2018). TVIs can provide invaluable guidance on necessary accommodations such as adjustments to lighting and materials. According to Fast (2018), children with visual impairments must learn through experience—by actively participating—in order to master a skill. TVIs can help classroom teachers plan instruction and provide accommodations to include young learners with visual impairments.

Similarly, teachers can collaborate with a specialist for Deaf and Hard of Hearing (DHH) to develop strategies to optimize the learning environment. These specialists assist the classroom teacher with techniques to reduce ambient noise levels and arrange seating to ensure that all students can fully engage during instruction (Taylor et al., 2020). These modifications are imperative for children with hearing impairments because they ensure better communication and understanding of academic content.

Speech-Language Pathologists (SLPs) are also vital partners to support language development. They provide approaches and interventions personalized to individual language needs, helping enhance communication skills and support academic achievement (Crais & Woods, 2016). SLPs contribute specialized knowledge and skills related to communication, language, speech, feeding, swallowing, and augmentative and alternative communication (Crais & Woods, 2016). Teachers can work with SLPs to modify materials for children with DD to ensure their active participation in the classroom.

Finally, a school nurse can be particularly helpful, especially for young children with chronic illnesses. Nurses conduct initial health evaluations to identify children who have chronic illnesses including asthma, diabetes, or epilepsy. They also dispense medication and are an important participant in developing Individualized Health Plans (IHPs). School nurses are prepared to respond to medical crises, particularly in children with chronic illness. They create and implement emergency response plans, as well as train teachers and staff on these procedures (Uhm et al., 2020).

Figure 3.6 provides a list of collaborative partners that many early childhood teachers work with to ensure inclusion for learners with DD and chronic illnesses. It is important to note this is not a comprehensive list. Teachers' abilities to access and collaborate with these professionals might be dependent on the setting (e.g., early childhood centers situated within public school divisions, standalone early childhood centers).

Working with Families and Caregivers

Perhaps the most important collaborative partner for an early childhood teacher is the family or caregiver. Families serve as an essential resource for early childhood educators, especially in comprehending and addressing the unique needs of each child. The Division for Early Childhood (DEC) emphasizes that parents and caregivers possess expert knowledge about their children due to their extensive and close involvement in

Teacher of the Visually Impaired (TVI)	• **Role:** Provides guidance on accommodations for visual impairments. • **Supports:** Adjustments to lighting, materials, and classroom environment.
Specialist for Deaf and Hard of Hearing (DHH)	• **Role:** Develops strategies for optimizing learning environments for hearing impairments. • **Supports:** Reducing ambient noise, optimal seating arrangements.
Speech-Language Pathologist (SLP)	• **Role:** Offers strategies for language development. • **Supports:** Techniques and interventions to improve communication skills.
Special Education Teacher	• **Role:** Provides expertise on instructional modifications and strategies. • **Supports:** Tailored instructional methods for learners with disabilities.
School Nurse	• **Role:** Addresses questions about feeding, medication, and nutrition. • **Supports:** Manages dietary needs, medical concerns.
Families/Caregivers	• **Role:** Shares insights and updates on child's needs and progress. • **Supports:** Information on preferences, routines, and changes in health.

Fig. 3.6 Collaborative partners to assist with instruction for inclusion

their care during non-school hours (DEC, 2014). This deep familiarity allows families to provide teachers with critical insights into what strategies and approaches work best for their child, particularly in managing medical and sensory needs. By sharing detailed information about their child's routines, preferences, and effective interventions, families enable teachers to tailor their practices to better support each child's development and well-being.

Moreover, maintaining open communication with families helps ensure that any changes in a child's medical or sensory needs are promptly addressed. Regular updates from families permit teachers to adapt their strategies and interventions as needed, fostering a cohesive approach to the child's care and education. Coordinated activities between home and school further enhance the consistency and effectiveness of support strategies, creating a seamless learning experience that bridges the gap between these two critical environments (DEC, 2014). In addition to DEC Recommended Practices, NAEYC emphasizes that family-centered practices involve respecting and valuing the family's role in their child's development and learning. This approach prioritizes building strong, collaborative relationships with families, recognizing them as the primary educators of their children and experts in their unique needs. By engaging in open dialogue and actively seeking family input, teachers can align classroom practices with the child's home experiences and preferences, ensuring a more holistic and individualized approach to education. Family-centered practices also encourage the adaptation of teaching methods to reflect the cultural, linguistic, and personal contexts of each child, thereby enhancing the relevance and effectiveness of educational interventions. According to a recent study by Sands and Meadan (2023), families need opportunities to share past experiences and build trusting relationships. By collaborating closely with families, teachers can form a more comprehensive and responsive educational plan that reflects each child's distinctive needs and promotes their overall growth.

Conclusion

It is important to remember that the child is a young learner first, and they are not defined by their disabilities or medical conditions. Therefore, a teacher's primary goal should be the same as it is for any other student—play, learn, and develop relationships. Academic content is no different. By utilizing practices of MTSS, UDL, and fostering collaborative relationships, early childhood teachers can ensure best practices for the inclusion of all young learners.

With that being said, there is a lack of sufficient research on using UDL and other strategies for this specific population and age group. More targeted studies are needed to explore any unanticipated benefits, as well as the potential challenges teachers may encounter when implementing these recommended practices for young children with DD and chronic illness. Additionally, factors such as coaching, funding, and available services in the setting must be considered to ensure effective implementation and support for educators working with these students. Understanding these factors is crucial for developing practical, evidence-based approaches that can be successfully integrated into classrooms.

Directions for Future Research, Policy, and Practice

All of the recommended practices in this chapter (e.g., MTSS, UDL, the Pyramid Model, NAEYC and DEC recommended practices) are known to promote effective inclusion of all children, but these practices may not be widely adopted or implemented as recommended in all early childhood education settings. Early childhood educators will need qualified coaches who can train, mentor, and support implementation of these strategies. More important than specific strategies, early childhood educators will need to know how, when, and with whom to implement these techniques. Each child will present a unique set of strengths and needs, therefore coaching and mentoring needs to focus on developing teachers as flexible problem solvers who have the skills needed to support all students in their classroom. Future research should investigate how coaching and mentoring in these areas increases teachers' confidence to support the inclusion of children with DD and chronic illness.

Author Note We would like to acknowledge our contributing student researchers: Ashley Edsall, Stacey Hammond, Alivia Palmer, and Shelley Gies.

References

Agyapong, B., Obuobi-Donkor, G., Burback, L., & Wei, Y. (2022). Stress, burnout, anxiety, and depression among teachers: A scoping review. *International Journal of Environmental Research and Public Health, 19*(17), 1–42. https://doi.org/10.3390/ijerph191710706

Allen, G. E., Common, E. A., Germer, K. A., Lane, K. L., Buckman, M. M., Oakes, W. P., & Menzies, H. M. (2019). A systematic review of the evidence base for active supervision in pre-K–12 settings. *Behavioral Disorders, 45*(3), 167–182. https://doi.org/10.1177/0198742919837646

Anderson, E. (2014). Examining interdisciplinary collaboration within a comprehensive early childhood education framework. *Head Start Dialogue, 17*(3), 1–15. https://doi.org/10.55370/hsdialog.v17i3.190

Artman-Meeker, A., Barton, E. E., Strain, P. S., & Hemmeter, M. L. (2021). Understanding, preventing, and responding to challenging behavior. In M. Hemmeter, M. Ostrosky, & L. Fox (Eds.), *Unpacking the pyramid model: A practical guide for preschool teachers* (pp. 16–23). Paul H. Brookes Publishing.

Bandura, A. (1997). *Self-efficacy: The exercise of control* (Vol. 604). Worth Publishers.

Barni, D., Danioni, F., & Benevene, P. (2019). Teachers' self-efficacy: The role of personal values and motivations for teaching. *Frontiers in Psychology, 10*, 1–7. https://doi.org/10.3389/fpsyg.2019.01645

Barrio, B. L., & Hollingshead, A. (2017). Reaching out to paraprofessionals: Engaging professional development aligned with the universal design for learning framework in rural communities. *Rural Special Education Quarterly, 36*(3), 136–145. https://doi.org/10.1177/8756870517721693

Barton, E., & Banerjee, R. (2013). Culturally responsive behavioral supports for children with challenging behavior and their families. In M. Ostrowsky & S. Sandall (Eds.), *Addressing young children's challenging behavior* (Young exceptional children monograph series no. 15) (pp. 59–75). Division of Early Childhood.

Benson-Goldberg, S., & Erickson, K. (2024). Reported and enacted emergent literacy instruction: Understanding young students with extensive support and complex communication needs, opportunity to learn. *Topics in Early Childhood Special Education, 44*(1), 6–19. https://doi.org/10.1177/02711214241235404

Carrington, S., Berthelsen, D., Nickerson, J., Nickerson, J. M., Walker, S., & Meldrum, K. (2016). Teachers' experiences of inclusion of children with developmental disabilities across the early years of school. *Journal of Psychologists and Counsellors in Schools, 26*(2), 139–154. https://doi.org/10.1017/jgc.2016.19

Carter, D. R., & Pool, J. L. (2012). Appropriate social behavior: Teaching expectations to young children. *Early Childhood Education Journal, 40*, 315–321. https://doi.org/10.1007/s10643-012-0516-y

Carver-Thomas, D., & Darling-Hammond, L. (2019). The trouble with teacher turnover: How teacher attrition affects students and schools. *Education Policy Analysis Archives, 27*(36). https://doi.org/10.14507/epaa.27.3699

Coleman, J. C., Crosby, M. G., Irwin, H. K., Dennis, L. R., Simpson, C. G., & Rose, C. A. (2012). Preventing challenging behaviors in preschool: Effective strategies for classroom teachers. *Young Exceptional Children, 16*(3), 3–10. https://doi.org/10.1177/1096250612464641

Crais, E. R., & Woods, J. (2016). The role of speech-language pathologists in providing early childhood special education. In B. Reichow, B. Boyd, E. Barton, & S. Odom (Eds.), *Handbook of early childhood special education* (pp. 1–20). Springer. https://doi.org/10.1007/978-3-319-28492-7_19

Darragh, H. (2007). Universal design for early childhood education: Ensuring access and equity for all. *Early Childhood Education Journal, 35*(2), 167–171. https://doi.org/10.1007/s10643-007-0177-4

DEC/NAEYC. (2009). Early childhood inclusion: A joint position statement of the Division for Early Childhood (DEC) and the National Association for the Education of Young Children (NAEYC). The University of North Carolina, FPG Child Development Institute.

Division for Early Childhood. (2014). *DEC recommended practices in early intervention/early childhood special education 2014.* http://www.dec-sped.org/dec-recommended-practices

Fast, D. K. (2018). Including children with visual impairments in the early childhood classroom. In D. Farland-Smith (Ed.), *Early childhood education* (pp. 123–137). InTechOpen. https://doi.org/10.5772/intechopen.80928

Fox, L., Hemmeter, M. L., Ostrosky, M., & Corso, R. (2021). Overview of the pyramid model. In M. Hemmeter, M. Ostrosky, & L. Fox (Eds.), *Unpacking the pyramid model: A practical guide for preschool teachers* (pp. 1–8). Paul H. Brookes Publishing.

Gauvreau, A. N., Lohmann, M. J., & Hovey, K. A. (2019). Using a universal design for learning framework to provide multiple means of representation in the early childhood classroom. *The Journal of Special Education Apprenticeship, 8*(1). https://doi.org/10.58729/2167-3454.1083

Greenwood, C. R., Carta, J. J., Schnitz, A. G., Irvin, D. W., Jia, F., & Atwater, J. (2019). Filling an information gap in preschool MTSS and RTI decision-making. *Exceptional Children, 85*(3), 271–290. https://doi.org/10.1177/0014402918812473

Gupta, S. S., Henninger, W. R., IV, & Vinh, M. E. (2014). *First steps to preschool inclusion: How to jumpstart your program-wide plan.* Paul H. Brookes Publishing.

Guralnick, M. J. (2011). Why early intervention works: A systems perspective. *Infants & Young Children, 24*(1), 6–28. https://doi.org/10.1097/IYC.0b013e3182002cfe

Hamre, B. K., & Pianta, R. C. (2004). Self-reported depression in non-familial caregivers: Prevalence and associations with caregiver behavior in child-care settings. *Early Childhood Research Quarterly, 19*(2), 297–318. https://doi.org/10.1016/j.ecresq.2004.04.006

Hamre, B. K., & Pianta, R. C. (2005). Can instructional and emotional support in the first-grade classroom make a difference for children at risk of school failure? *Child Development, 76*(5), 949–967. https://doi.org/10.1111/j.1467-8624.2005.00889.x

Hemmeter, M. L., Ostrosky, M. M., & Corso, R. M. (2012). Preventing and addressing challenging behavior: Common questions and practical strategies. *Young Exceptional Children, 15*(2), 32–46. https://doi.org/10.1177/1096250611427350

Hunt, P., Soto, G., Maier, J., Liboiron, N., & Bae, S. (2004). Collaborative teaming to support preschoolers with severe disabilities who are placed in general education early childhood programs. *Topics in Early Childhood Special Education, 24*(3), 123–142. https://doi.org/10.1177/02711214040240030101

Individuals with Disabilities Education Improvement Act of 2004, Pub. L. No. 101–476, 20 U.S.C. §§ 1400 et seq.

Jennings, P. A., & Greenberg, M. T. (2009). The prosocial classroom: Teacher social and emotional competence in relation to student and classroom outcomes. *Review of Educational Research, 79*(1), 491–525. https://doi.org/10.3102/0034654308325693

Klassen, R., & Chiu, M. M. (2010). Effects on teachers' self-efficacy and job satisfaction: Teacher gender, years of experience, and job stress. *Journal of Educational Psychology, 102*(3), 741–756. https://doi.org/10.1037/a0019237

Kwon, K. A., Jeon, S., Jeon, L., & Castle, S. (2019). The role of teachers' depressive symptoms in classroom quality and child developmental outcomes in Early Head Start programs. *Learning and Individual Differences, 74*, 1–13. https://doi.org/10.1016/j.lindif.2019.06.002

Mashburn, A. J., Pianta, R. C., Hamre, B. K., Downer, J. T., Barbarin, O. A., Bryant, D., et al. (2008). Measures of classroom quality in prekindergarten and children's development of academic, language, and social skills. *Child Development, 79*, 732–749. https://doi.org/10.1111/j.1467-8624.2008.01154.x

McCormick, M. P., O'Connor, E. E., Cappella, E., & McClowry, S. G. (2013). Teacher-child relationships and academic achievement: A multilevel propensity score model approach. *Journal of School Psychology, 51*(5), 611–624. https://doi.org/10.1016/j.jsp.2013.05.001

Miedema, S. T., Brian, A., Pennell, A., Liberman, L., True, L., Webster, C., & Stodden, D. (2022). The effects of an integrative, universally designed motor skill intervention for young children with and without disabilities. *Adapted Physical Activity Quarterly, 39*(2), 179–196. https://doi.org/10.1123/apaq.2021-0031

Mortensen, J. A., & Barnett, M. A. (2014). Teacher–child interactions in infant/toddler child care and socioemotional development. *Early Education and Development, 26*(2), 209–229. https://doi.org/10.1080/10409289.2015.985878

National Association for the Education of Young Children (NAEYC). (2009a). *NAEYC standards for early childhood professional preparation: Position statement.* Author.

National Association for the Education of Young Children. (2009b). *Developmentally appropriate practice in early childhood programs serving children from birth through age 8: A position statement of the National Association for the Education of Young Children.*

National Center for Pyramid Model Interventions. (2021). *Preparing the pyramid: Classroom essentials.* https://challengingbehavior.org/docs/Preparing-for-the-Pyramid.pdf

Navaitienė, J., & Stasiūnaitienė, E. (2021). The goal of the universal design for learning: Development of all to expert learners. In A. Galkienė & O. Monkevičienė (Eds.), *Improving inclusive education through universal design for learning: Inclusive learning and educational equity* (pp. 17–36). Springer. https://doi.org/10.1007/978-3-030-80658-3_2

Ngyuen, T., Ansari, A., Pianta, R. C., Whittaker, J. V., Vitiello, V. E., & Ruznek, E. (2020). The classroom relational environment and children's early development in preschool. *Social Development, 29*(4). https://doi.org/10.1111/sode.12447

O'Connor, E., & McCartney, K. (2007). Examining teacher-student relationships and achievement as part of an ecological model of development. *American Educational Research Journal, 44*(2), 340–369. https://doi.org/10.3102/0002831207302172

Palacios, N. (2017). Why all teachers matter: The relationship between long-term teacher and classroom quality and children's reading achievement. *Journal of Research in Childhood Education, 31*(2), 178–198. https://doi.org/10.1080/02568543.2016.1272509

Price, C. L., & Steed, E. A. (2016). Culturally responsive strategies to support young children with challenging behavior. *YC Young Children, 71*(5), 36–43.

Rappolt-Schlichtmann, G., Daley, S. G., Lim, S., Lapinski, S., Robinson, K. H., & Johnson, M. (2013). Universal design for learning and elementary school science: Exploring the efficacy, use, and perceptions of a web-based science notebook. *Journal of Educational Psychology, 105*(4), 1210–1225. https://doi.org/10.1037/a0033217

Rausch, A., & Strain, P. (2021). Why focus on quality inclusion as part of a statewide Pyramid Model implementation? *National Center for Pyramid Model Innovations.* https://challengingbehavior.org/docs/Why-quality-inclusion_whitepaper.pdf

Sands, M. M., & Meadan, H. (2023). Transition to kindergarten for children with disabilities: Parent and kindergarten teacher perceptions and experiences. *Topics in Early Childhood Special Education, 43*(4), 265–277. https://doi.org/10.1177/02711214221146748

Shepley, C., & Grisham-Brown, J. (2019). Multi-tiered systems of support for preschool-aged children: A review and meta-analysis. *Early Childhood Research Quarterly, 47*, 296–308. https://doi.org/10.1016/j.ecresq.2019.01.004

Sutton, R. E., & Wheatley, K. F. (2003). Teachers' emotions and teaching: A review of the literature and directions for future research. *Educational Psychology Review, 15*(4), 327–358. https://doi.org/10.1023/A:1026131715856

Taylor, K., Neild, R., & Fitzpatrick, M. (2020). Universal design for learning: Promoting access in early childhood education for deaf and hard of hearing children. *Perspectives on Early Childhood Psychology and Education, 5*(2), 75–91. https://doi.org/10.58948/2834-8257.1059

Thomas, E. R., Lembke, E. S., & Gandhi, A. G. (2023). Universal design for learning within an integrated multitiered system of support. *Learning Disabilities Research & Practice, 38*(1), 57–69. https://doi.org/10.1111/ldrp.12302

Tschannen-Moran, M., & Hoy, A. W. (2001). Teacher efficacy: Capturing an elusive construct. *Teaching and Teacher Education, 17*(7), 783–805. https://doi.org/10.1016/S0742-051X(01)00036-1

UDL and Multi-Tiered Systems of Supports (MTSS). (n.d.). *SST6.* https://www.sst6.org/UDLandMulti-TieredSystemsofSupportsMTSS.aspx

Uhm, J. Y., Choi, M. Y., & Lee, H. (2020). School nurses' perceptions regarding barriers and facilitators in caring for children with chronic diseases in school settings: A mixed studies review. *Nursing & Health Sciences, 22*(4), 868–880. https://doi.org/10.1111/nhs.12786

Wang, M. T., & Eccles, J. S. (2012). Social support matters: Longitudinal effects of social support on three dimensions of school engagement from middle to high school. *Child Development, 83*(3), 877–895. https://doi.org/10.1111/j.1467-8624.2012.01745.x

Wentzel, K. R., & Brophy, J. E. (2013). *Motivating students to learn* (4th ed.). Routledge. https://doi.org/10.4324/9780203108017

Chapter 4
Playground Design and Activities to Foster Inclusion of Children with Developmental Disabilities

Tina L. Stanton-Chapman

Abstract This chapter analyzes the design, implementation, and impact of playgrounds that foster inclusion for young children with developmental disabilities. It highlights the rising prevalence of these disabilities in the U.S. and the importance of social participation—engagement with environment and peers—for children's well-being. Differentiating accessible, inclusive, and universal playgrounds, the chapter emphasizes that universal playgrounds, based on Universal Design principles, best serve children and caregivers of all abilities with equitable, engaging, and developmentally appropriate play. Using evidence-based design and stakeholder feedback, a case study of a universally designed playground shows high utilization across ages, with over 80% of the facility accessible. Survey and observational data reveal positive experiences for children, grandparents, and caregivers, including shared play and increased engagement. While barriers to social play persist, universal playgrounds help overcome exclusion, supporting social integration for children with disabilities. The chapter advocates for data-driven evaluation and inclusive playground design to fulfill the rights and needs of diverse families.

Keywords Young children with developmental disabilities · Playground design · Inclusion · Accessible playgrounds · Universal playgrounds

Playground Design and Activities to Foster Inclusion of Children with Developmental Disabilities

In the United States, the percentage of children with a developmental disability increased from 3.9% in 2008 to 4.3% in 2019 (Young, 2021). This 4.3% represents an estimated 2.6 million households who have at least one child in the home with a

T. L. Stanton-Chapman (✉)
Elementary Education and Human Development, College of Education, Criminal Justice, Human Services, and Information Technology, University of Cincinnati, Cincinnati, OH, USA
e-mail: stantot@ucmail.uc.edu

L. Nabors and T. Stanton-Chapman (eds.), *Developmental Disabilities and Chronic Illness in Young Children*, Springer Series on Child and Family Studies,
https://doi.org/10.1007/978-3-032-08523-8_4

disability (U. S. Census Bureau 2019). Article 19 of the Convention on the Rights of Persons with Disabilities (Department of Economic and Social Affairs Disability, 2024) states that all persons with disabilities have the right to live in a community with choices equal to others. Despite the right for equal participation in the community, caregivers, who have children with disabilities, reported that their children could not socially participate on a playground (Stanton-Chapman & Schmidt, 2019). Social participation refers to an individual's ability to engage with the physical environment and interact with others who are in that environment at the same time (Levasseur et al., 2022). In a study examining the social participation of children with disabilities on playgrounds, caregivers reported one of three options: (a) their child with a disability stayed home while other family members participated in outdoor play, (b) the family drove over 30-min from their home to locate more inclusive playground facilities, and/or (c) the family participated in activities at home (e.g., board games) (Stanton-Chapman & Schmidt, 2018). Special education professionals (e.g., teachers, occupational therapists, physical therapists) not only corroborated these results, but also highlighted (a) the need for a playground environment that meets the needs of *all* children, (b) the segregation that takes place on a playground between children with and without disabilities, and (c) the lack of interest in accessible playgrounds in children of all abilities.

Playground Types

The ADA Accessibility Guidelines for Play Areas (2000) and the ADA Standards for Accessible Design (2010) advocate for full social participation of children with disabilities on playgrounds. While these guidelines and standards are helpful, playground manufacturers only have to ensure that accessibility standards are met in their playground equipment, but they do not have to provide evidence that *all* children are able to fully use this equipment, have an interest in using it, or ensure that the playground equipment has play value (Stanton-Chapman & Schmidt, 2016). Rather, the purpose of the accessibility guidelines is (a) to provide children who require the use of mobility devices (e.g., walkers, wheelchairs) access to the playground equipment and (b) to reduce life-threatening and deliberating injuries across all children (U. S. Architectural and Transportation Barriers Compliance Board, 2004).

The physical environment is thought to be a critical factor in children's development and play (Stanton-Chapman & Schmidt, 2019). The correlation between children's play environments and their overall well-being is best described using Gibson's Theory of Affordances (Gibson, 1950). In the Theory of Affordances, the affordances of the physical environment are what the environment offers the child and the complementary relationship between the child and the environment. Playgrounds offer multiple affordances and play behaviors to children such as running-on, running-off, swinging on, and swinging off, climbing on, and climbing off (Sandseter, 2009). They also provide potential play partners who may socially interact with the child.

Accessible Playgrounds In 2019, Stanton-Chapman and Schmidt provided a summary of the three different types of playgrounds. The first type of playground is an *accessible playground*. Accessible playgrounds meet the minimum requirements that are required by law for playground development for children with disabilities. The affordances of an accessible playground include (a) providing ramps leading to upper decks and/or provide transfer stations, (b) providing ground level activities and elevated activities (if required), and (c) providing no barriers to the entrance or along the play structure's pathways. Although children, who use mobility devices, are given access to the upper deck of the playground structure, there are limited play activities on the play deck. Typically, the upper deck offers activity panels, but these activity panels tend to be uninteresting to children or provide sensory activities that are outside the arm reach of children with physical disabilities (Stanton-Chapman & Schmidt, 2018). Furthermore, many children who use mobility devices are unable to use the slides without adult assistance (Boundless Playgrounds, 2010). As a result, children, who use wheelchairs, may watch their peers go down the slides or climb a pole while they cannot. This has the potential to impact the children's social participation.

Figure 4.1 depicts an accessible playground. The black arrow points to a transfer station. A transfer station provides access to the elevated play components of a playground structure. A child in a wheelchair might use this structure, wheeling over to the transfer station where they climb out of their wheelchair and either crawl or walk up the play structure. The pink arrow points to a ground level activity (i.e., drums). A child, who uses a wheelchair, can wheel over to the drums and play them. Finally, the playground structure is surrounded by mulch to provide open access. Mulch is an acceptable surfacing material for mobility devices on a playground setting.

Inclusive Playgrounds The second type of playground is an *inclusive playground.* Inclusive playgrounds meet the accessible playground affordances plus (a) provide play equipment that challenges children at various ability levels, (b) provide extra-wide travel routes, and (c) provide safety surfacing that allows children with mobility devices access to all areas of the playground. Inclusive playgrounds allow children with disabilities to play alongside their peers; however, they also have limitations. First, they are typically designed with a child's specific disability in mind (Stanton-Chapman & Schmidt, 2018). For example, Preston's Hope Playground (https://www.prestonshope.com/) was designed for a child born with spinal muscular atrophy so he could socially participate with his peers on a community playground. Such playgrounds typically work while the target child is within the developmental age range of the facility, but the target child eventually ages out of the playground. Once the target child ages out of the playground, many communities report that the playground no longer meets the community's needs (Stanton-Chapman & Schmidt, 2018). Second, inclusive playgrounds tend to be expensive and communities need to fundraise to meet the expense. Fundraising efforts take considerable time, and thus, communities find that the target child, for whom the inclusive playground is designed and built, ages out or passes away (McConkey, 2018). Finally, many children without

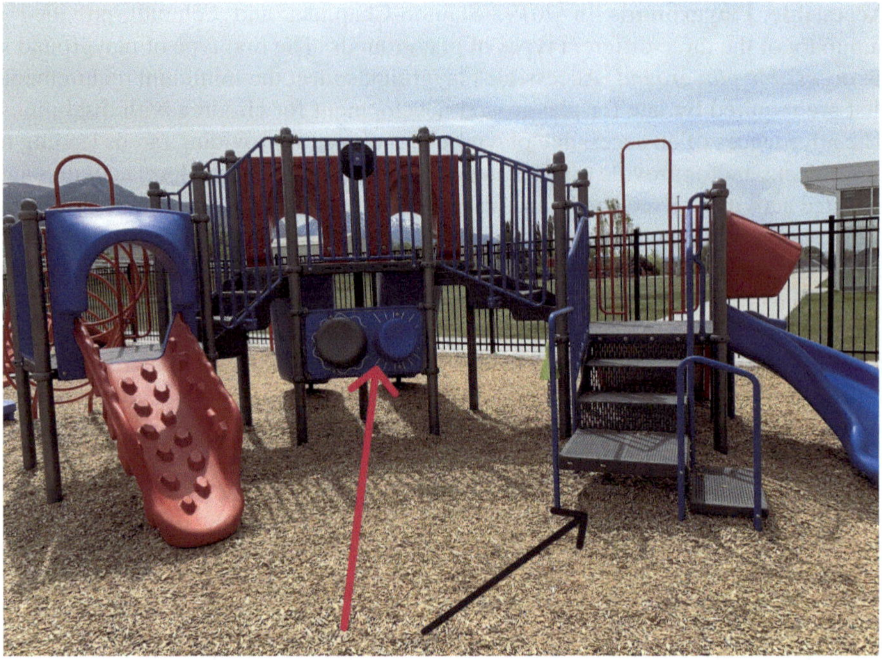

Fig. 4.1 Picture of an accessible playground

disabilities do not find inclusive playgrounds fun and engaging due to the disability focus of the playground (Stanton-Chapman & Schmidt, 2016).

Figure 4.2 depicts an inclusive playground. This playground has multiple play activities (e.g., playground structure with ramps, a swing structure, a climbing structure) for children with disabilities. The main play structure has extra-wide ramps (yellow arrow) to provide ample access to the elevated areas. Children, who use mobility devices, do not have to leave their wheelchairs or walkers behind to play on the playground structure. This playground also uses pour-in-place safety surfacing (black arrow) rather than mulch. Pour-in-place (PIP) safety surfacing typically consists of colorful crumb rubber held together by a binding agent that creates a seamless, unitary playground surface. PIP allows wheelchairs, walkers, and strollers to maneuver throughout the play area with little difficulty.

Universal Playgrounds The third type of playground is a *universal playground.* A universal playground is one that meets the Principles of Universal Design—where every child regardless of gender, race/ethnicity, age, or ability or disability is welcomed and benefits physically, developmentally, and socially (Center for Universal Design, 1997). Universal playgrounds meet the accessible and inclusive affordances plus (a) play equipment is of appropriate size and space. Children can approach, reach, manipulate, and use the equipment regardless of body size, posture, or mobility, (b) the design does not disadvantage or stigmatize any groups of users,

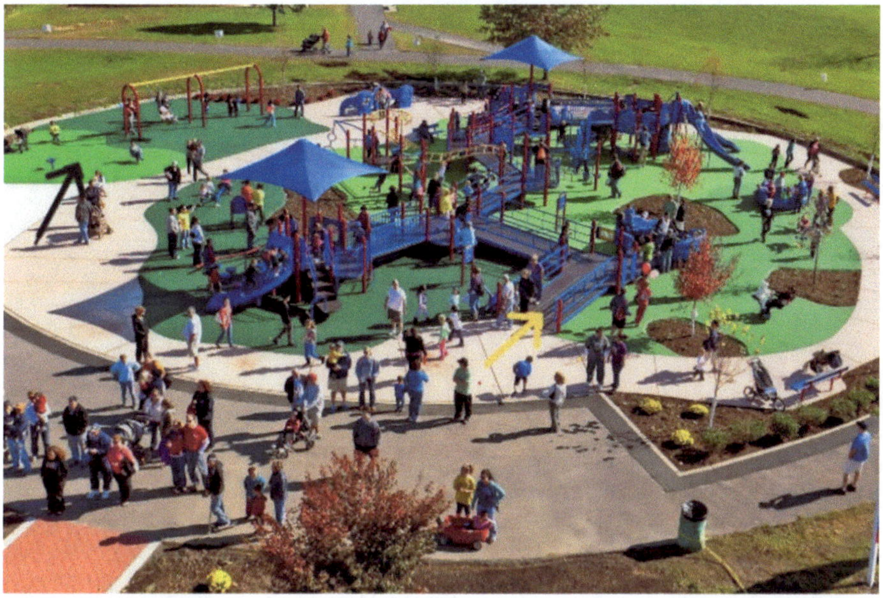

Fig. 4.2 Picture of an inclusive playground

(c) the design accommodates a wide-range of individual preferences and abilities, (d) the design is easy to understand regardless of the user's abilities, and (e) the design can be efficiently used with little fatigue.

Figure 4.3 provides an example of a playground that adheres to the Principles of Universal Design. Results from Stanton-Chapman and Schmidt (2016, 2017, 2018) were collated to inform the design of this playground. The goal was to develop a playground that was evidence-based (e.g., built based on recommendations from research), met the needs of children of varying ages and abilities, held children's interest for a minimum of 30 min, and was designed in such a way that it would not appear to be a playground for children with disabilities. Over 80% of the overall playground facility is accessible to *all* individuals. When designing the playground, the best equipment from multiple playground manufacturing companies was used rather than playground equipment from one playground manufacturer, which is typical for playground design. Playground equipment that is developmentally appropriate for infants to 12 years was incorporated into the overall design. Given that the playground is over 80% ground level, grandparents and caregivers with disabilities can be in close proximity to their children and may participate in their play, if desired. The playground encompasses seven play zones—an infant and toddler play area, musical instruments, a sensory maze, a turf hill with metal slides and tunnels, a mega tower for climbing and sliding, a zipline, traditional swings, and an accelerator swing. A thorough description of each play zone appears in Stanton-Chapman and Schmidt (2017).

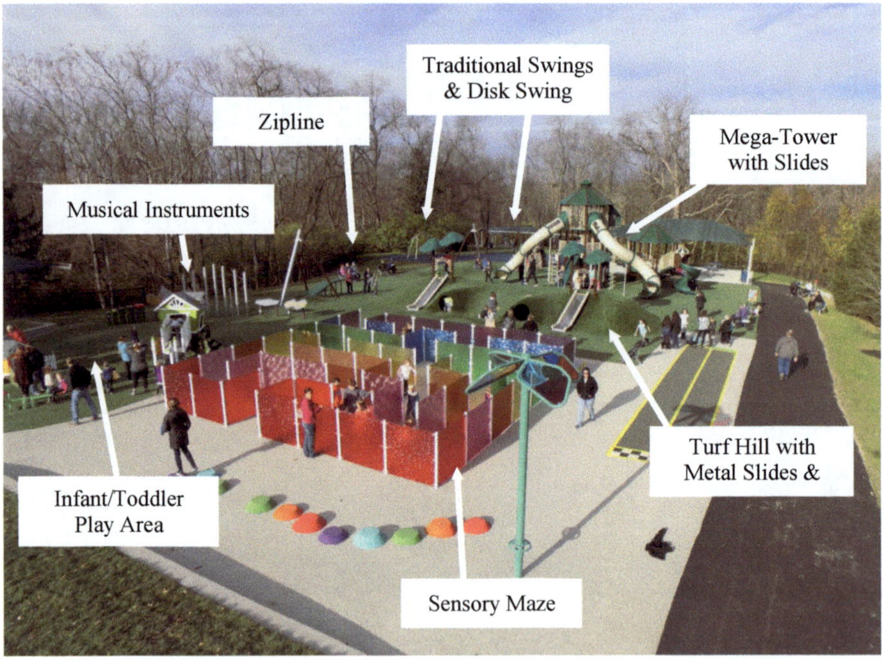

Fig. 4.3 Picture of a universal playground

Data-Driven Evaluation of a Universally Designed Playground

Data drove the creation, build, implementation, and evaluation of the universally designed playground (Stanton-Chapman & Schmidt, 2016, 2017, 2018). After the playground opened, data were collected at the three levels—adults, children, and observations of children and adults at the playground to understand use of the playground and stakeholder evaluation of the playground areas and play in this unique setting. The development of data collection tools and results from using these tools to assess use of play areas and perceptions of the playground are presented in the following sections of this chapter.

Data Collection Tools

Adult Surveys

Individuals who visited the universally designed playground were surveyed from January 2018 to March 2023. Any adult, 18 years and older, who visited the playground at least one time from when the playground opened in October 2017, was invited to participate in an online survey. The survey asked: (a) demographic questions about survey respondents and their families (e.g., number of children in the family, ages of family members, disability status of family members), (b) information regarding their visits, length of stay, playground zones visited, and (c) information regarding their child's most and least liked playground zones and playground equipment. Invitations to participate in the online survey were done through social media outlets, a local story in the city and community newspapers, a link on the community's government page, and flyers given to local childcare centers and elementary schools. The invitations described the study as a research project examining their thoughts on the playground.

Adult Open-Ended Survey Questions

All adult respondents were invited to answer several open-ended questions once they concluded the online survey. The open-ended questions varied from "*how would you change or improve the playground?*" to "*did you participate in play with your children and/or grandchildren while visiting the playground? If yes, what activities did you do together?*" Adult participants were not required to answer the questions. They had the option to conclude the survey without answering the open-ended questions. The open-ended survey questions required answers to be typed into the response boxes. None of the respondents could be identified by their narrative responses.

Child Survey

In April 2018, the principals of these three elementary schools located within 5 miles of the playground were contacted for participation. The principals were asked if paper-based surveys could be distributed to all pre-kindergarten through sixth grade students within their schools. All three principals granted permission for the survey to be conducted in their school.

There were two versions of the child survey—a pre-kindergarten through first grade survey and a second grade through sixth grade survey. The surveys asked the same questions, but differed in readability, response format, and how the surveys were delivered. An early childhood literacy expert, with over 25 years of university experience, reviewed the two surveys and provided feedback on readability across the various ages. Surveys were revised based on the expert's feedback. The pre-kindergarten through first grade survey posed questions that were within the reading levels of 5-to-7-year-old children. Teachers read the survey to their students, one question at a time. Students answered by circling a happy face if they agreed with the statement or a sad face if they disagreed with the statement. The second grade through sixth grade survey posed questions that were within the reading levels of 8-to-9-year-olds. Students completed the surveys, on their own, during the school day. Students answered by circling "yes" if they agreed with the statement or "no" if they disagreed with the statement. Each survey contained 15 questions including demographic (e.g., grade, age), questions with pictures of playground equipment asking the child if they played in the area pictured, a question where the child is asked to draw an X on the picture where they played the least, and a question where the child is asked to circle their favorite play area and piece of playground equipment.

Direct Observations of Children Playing at the Playground

Direct observations of children playing at the playground were conducted from March through October in 2018, 2019, and 2021. Observations were conducted on weekdays and weekends during morning, afternoon, and evenings from 8:00 AM to 8:00 PM. Observations were counterbalanced so that there were equal numbers of weekday and weekend observations across equal numbers of morning, afternoon, and evening observations. Observers collected data in two-hour time increments, broken into 10-min intervals.

The Destination Playground Frequency Observation Code (Stanton-Chapman & Rhoades, 2018) was used to code observations at the playground. This code measures the number of boys and girls in a playground zone, within a specified time interval. The coder counts the number of boys and girls present in the specified zone using momentary interval coding. All coding sessions began at the top of the hour and continued for 2 h. At the beginning of the observation, the coder started the 10-min interval in Zone 1 and proceeded through the zones, in order, counting the number of boys and girls in each zone. All zones were visited in the 10-min interval. Once a 10-min interval was completed, the next interval began and the coder proceeded through the zones, in order, following the same procedures until the 2 h were completed.

The observational manual outlined the exact travel paths coders were required to follow as they counted boys and girls. Pictures of each zone were provided. A green X indicated where the coder entered the zone and began counting. Red arrows indicated the expected walking path taken by the coder through the zone. A red X indicated where the coder stopped counting in the zone.

Description of Coders All observations were conducted by an early childhood education professor and graduate students. Coders did not wear identifying clothing or name badges and attempted to blend into the community as they coded.

Description of Coder Training and Reliability Coding Reliability observations were equally distributed across type of day (weekend, weekday) and time of day (morning, afternoon, evening). Using a computer-based program (MOOSES, Tapp, 2021), a sequential comparison of the coded data was made on a point-by-point basis. The program recorded an agreement if both coders counted the number of boys or girls in a play zone within two. For example, if the primary coder said there were four girls in Zone 1 and the reliability coder said there were six in Zone 1, an agreement would be scored. The program recorded a disagreement if the coders differed in their frequency counts of boys and girls in a play zone by three or more. For example, if the primary coder said there were 10 boys in Zone 4 and the reliability coder said there were 13 boys in Zone 4, a disagreement would be scored. This reliability coding system was established because children were always on the move as the coders counted the children. Since the primary coder and the reliability coder did not discuss during the observations, they did not establish which boy or girl needed to be coded first. On any given day, at this playground, there could be 10 or more children in a zone, not including the adults. The within-two rule allowed for a small amount of error. Reliability was assessed using an exact agreement formula in which the total number of agreements was divided by the total number of agreements plus disagreements and multiplied by 100. To account for chance agreement, Cohen's (1960) kappa was calculated. Fleiss (1981) characterized kappa values: 0.40–0.60 (fair), 0.60–0.75 (good), and greater than 0.75 (excellent).

Results from Surveys and Observations Assessing the Universally Designed Playground

In this section, published and unpublished data regarding the universal playground is discussed by data collection method.

Adult Surveys

For all adult surveys, inclusionary criteria included: (a) an adult who is 18 years of age or older, (b) must have visited the universal playground in question at least one time with a child, (c) the visit must have occurred within the specified timeline, (d) the child who visited the playground with the adult must be between the ages of 6-month to 12-year in age, and (e) the adult must have a valid email address. A total of 948 adults responded to and completed the entire survey. Forty-one individuals opened the link to the survey but did not complete the entire survey. Their responses were not included in the final analyses. The overall response was: (a) 907 adults who opened the link to the online survey, (b) 96% who opened the link to the online survey successfully completed the entire survey, and (c) 4% who opened the link to the online survey but did not successfully complete the entire survey. All adults and

Table 4.1 Age range of the children brought to the playground

Age range	Number of children	Percentage
Birth to 2 years	398	22%
3–4 years	425	24%
5–7 years	628	35%
8–12 years	301	17%
13 years or older	52	2%
Total	1804	100%

their responses were kept anonymous. Although participants were required to enter their email address at the beginning of the survey, email addresses were not tied to data. Rather, email addresses ensured that respondents completed the online survey only once with a valid email address.

For the adult surveys, respondents varied in terms of their role: 610 (67%) described themselves as mothers, 164 (18%) as a grandparent, 91 (10%) as fathers, 28 (3%) as an aunt/uncle, 13 (1%) as an adult sibling, and 9 (1%) as a foster parent. Respondents were primarily female (771, 85%). For race/ethnicity, respondents also varied with 487 (54%) describing themselves as Caucasian, 137 (15%) as two or more races, 136 (15%) as African American, 115 (12%) as Hispanic or Latino/Latina, and 32 (4%) as Asian. Respondents were primarily in the 25-to-44 age bracket (584, 64%).

Table 4.1 presents the age range of the children brought to the playground. Because the respondents typically took more than one child to the playground, the total number of children exceeded the number of adults.

Of the 1804 children that the respondents brought to the playground, 91 (5%) children were reported as having a disability. Specific disability categories are reported in Table 4.2.

Table 4.2 Disability categories of children who visited the playground

Disability category	Number of children	Percentage
Autism	34	38%
Behavior disorder	1	1%
Developmental delay	5	5%
Hearing impairment	1	1%
Intellectual disability	1	1%
Learning disability	18	20%
Orthopedic impairment	2	2%
Sensory processing disorder	16	18%
Specific language impairment	13	13%
Visual impairment	1	1%
Total	91	100%

Table 4.3 Average time respondents reported playing at the playground

Average number of minutes	Number of respondents	Percentage
61 or more minutes	243	34%
46–60 min	301	43%
31–45 min	119	17%
16–30 min	38	5%
1–15 min	6	1%
Total	707	100%

Table 4.3 presents the average time respondents reported playing at the playground.

Adult Open-Ended Survey Questions

The open-ended survey questions required respondents to type their answers into response boxes. None of the respondents could be identified by their responses. Of the 907 respondents who participated in the adult survey, 747 (82%) respondents completed the open-ended survey. The remaining 160 (18%) individuals did not complete the open-ended survey.

Stanton-Chapman and Nabors (2024) published a study regarding grandparents and the universal playground. In it, many grandparents reported that they visited the playground 7-to-9 times within the given time period, and they visited 45-min or longer. In general, grandparents indicated that they brought grandchildren ages 6-month to 4-year and that they participated in play with their grandchildren. Play activities included swinging activities (e.g., swinging next to their grandchildren on a swing), running and hide-and-seek activities (e.g., child hides while the grandparent finds them; the grandparent and grandchild racing one another), and playground equipment activities (e.g., making music together in the musical instrument area, playing within the sensory maze). An open-ended survey question asked, "*what pieces of playground equipment did your child/grandchild use that you could not and why?*" Responses were grouped into four categories: (a) grandparent cannot physically use the playground equipment pieces due to age or ability, (b) grandchild was old enough to play alone on the playground equipment without an adult, (c) grandchild was playing with a peer or sibling, and (d) grandparents' adaptive equipment prevented them from using the playground equipment. Another open-ended survey question asked, "*what benefits, if any, do you receive from the universally designed playground?*" Examples of answers included "*I can play with my granddaughter instead of just watching her play,*" and "*it has an area for toddlers to play.*" The results from this study demonstrated that grandparents and grandchildren played together on the universal playground and both parties reaped positive affordances from the playground.

Stanton-Chapman, Rhoades, and Schmidt (2023) examined adult and child perceptions of the universal playground's sensory maze. To address the sensory needs of children and a literature and practice gap, the authors designed and built an outdoor sensory maze for use on playgrounds. One question asked in this study was "*what makes the playground unique in comparison to other playgrounds the respondents have visited with their children?*" Answers to this question centered around four themes: (a) the sensory maze provided sensory activities to children with sensory needs, (b) the sensory maze promoted creative play and built imagination, (c) the sensory maze was aesthetically pleasing and brightened up the playground, and (d) how the sensory maze allowed play across the age span and encouraged group play. The sensory maze was a favorite for children with sensory disabilities according to child surveys. Prior research has indicated that sensory playground equipment is not only needed for children with sensory disabilities, but such equipment can change the type of play children with disabilities elicit on a playground environment (Stanton-Chapman & Schmidt, 2016, 2017).

Child Surveys

For all child surveys, inclusionary criteria included: (a) a child who is enrolled at a public or private elementary school within 5 miles of the playground, (b) the child must be in a pre-kindergarten through sixth grade classroom within the elementary school, and (c) the child must have visited the playground at least one time within the specified timeline. A total of 881 children completed the survey. All children and their responses were kept anonymous as children did not put their names on the survey.

For the child surveys, 465 boys (53%) and 416 girls (47%) completed the survey. Respondents included 23 (3%) 4-year-olds, 33 (4%) 5-year-olds, 138 (16%) 6-year-olds, 134 (15%) 7-year-olds, 127 (14%) 8-year-olds, 116 (13%) 9-year-olds, 113 (13%) 10-year-olds, 120 (14%) 11-year-olds, and 77 (8%) 12-year-olds. Race/ethnicity and disability status data were not collected.

Children were asked to indicate their favorite playground zone by circling the picture which best depicts their selection. Across ages, the boys' top three choices were the mega tower 134 (29%) respondents, the zipline 127 (27%) respondents, and the turf hill 117 (25%) respondents. Girls' top three choices were the zipline 157 (38%) respondents, the turf hill 136 (33%) respondents, and the mega tower 88 (21%) respondents.

Children were asked to indicate their *least* favorite playground zone by marking an X on the picture which best depicts their selection. Across ages, the boys' top three choices for least favorite area were the infant/toddler area 189 (41%) respondents, the musical instruments 151 (32%) respondents, and the traditional swings 75 (16%) respondents. Girls' top three choices were the musical instruments 118 (28%) respondents, the traditional swings 101 (24%) respondents, and the disk swing 89 (21%) respondents.

Child Observations

Direct observations of children playing at the playground were conducted between March and October across 3 years. Frequency counts resulted in observations of 21,763 children. Due to the structure of the observations, children were most likely counted multiple times within the two-hour observations as the focus centered on *where* children played rather than *how many* children played at the playground. Of the 21,763 children, 10,534 were boys and 11,229 were girls. Age, disability status, and race/ethnicity were not coded during these observations due to Institutional Review Board (IRB) restrictions.

Boys tended to play in the mega tower zone ($n = 2904$), the turf hill zone ($n = 2078$), the zipline zone ($n = 1827$), and the sensory maze zone ($n = 1337$). Girls tended to play in the zipline zone (N = 2830), the mega tower zone (N = 2281), the turf hill zone (N = 1693), and the sensory maze zone (N = 1547). Overall, children played in the mega tower zone (N = 5185), the zipline zone (N = 4657), the turf hill zone (N = 3771), and the sensory maze zone (N = 2884) the most. These data coincide with the child survey data and demonstrate that children play where they said they played.

Boys tended to play the least in the disk swing zone (N = 277), the musical instrument zone (N = 366), and the traditional swing zone (N = 514). Girls tended to play the least in the musical instrument zone (N = 400), the disk swing zone (N = 418), and the traditional swing zone (N = 744). Overall, the least played in zones were the disk swing (N = 695), the musical instruments (N = 766), and the traditional swings (N = 1258).

The infant/toddler zone was visited by 1231 boys and 1316 girls for a total of 2547 children. According to qualitative notes taken by observational coders, the infant/toddler zone tended to be "policed" by caregivers. Caregivers were vocal in keeping older children out of the zone for safety purposes. These findings are reflected in the child survey data in that the infant/toddler zone was not selected as a most favorite play zone.

Stanton-Chapman, Schmidt, Rhoades, and Monnin (2020) explored the outcomes of a universally playground on child's play and compared these findings to an inclusive playground and its impact on children's play. The total number of 10-min observations across the two playgrounds was 18,794. The inclusive playground had 15-boys and 8-girls playing at the facility over the 6-month period. The average time spent on this playground was 15 min. While the playground had four distinct play zones, the 23 children only played on the large play structure. The universal playground had 10,534 boys and 11,229 girls playing at the facility over the 6-month period. The average time at this facility was 1-h, 15-min. Given that so few children played on the inclusive playground, direct comparisons between the two playgrounds could not be made. The results obtained from this study emphasized what caregivers, teachers, and children have already told us—accessible and inclusive playgrounds are boring, uninteresting, and have limited play and social value for children.

In a second observational study, Stanton-Chapman and Schmidt (2021) examined the social play behaviors of the same six participants on a school and a community playground. The participants were observed for five 30-min observations on a school playground and for five 30-min observations on a community playground. Results indicated that children's play skill competence varies by setting. Specifically, children demonstrated higher levels of associative and cooperative play on the school playground but higher levels of solitary and parallel play on the community playground. The difference in play styles by playground appears to be a function of available play partners and children not feeling comfortable playing with children they do not know. It is possible that children use parallel and onlooker play as a means of getting more comfortable with unfamiliar children with the hope of receiving an initiating play bid. The knowledge from this study suggests to playground manufacturers that associative and cooperative play does not magically happen due to the presence of playground equipment, but rather to the peer relationships that children have with others on the playground setting.

Economic Value of the Playground to the Community

The public value of a playground is defined as the economic value a playground brings to its local community (Meynhardt, 2009). The *proximate principle of a playground* is defined as the positive impact on property values that a playground may provide to a community (Crompton, 2001). This principle is based on the observation that people are frequently willing to pay a larger amount of money for a home close to the playground. A determining factor of a playground's impact on property values is the extent of the playground's circumference (Little, 1990). Playgrounds with a larger circumference have a larger edge—the number of homes and residences adjacent to the playground (Crompton, 2001).

The edge of the universal playground is home residences built in the 1980s. According to the county auditor's database, property values for the seven roads forming the playground's circumference increased by 4.8% between 11/01/2017 and 12/31/2020. This value demonstrates the proximate principle of the playground. Between 01/01/2014 and 10/31/2017, property values for these roads ranged from \$110,000 to \$255,000. Between 11/01/2017 and 12/31/2020, property values for these roads ranged from \$165,000 to \$340,000. This time period is after the opening of the playground and the housing bubble that started in 2021. After the housing bubble in 2021 (01/01/2021–07/31/2023), property values for these roads ranged from \$200,000 to \$350,000.

Urban planners and public space designers often wish to understand and observe who is utilizing a playground. This information is a playground's outreach (Moran et al., 2019). Playground outreach may be calculated using many different methods (e.g., surveying playground patrons, observing the demographic characteristics of playground patrons). The playground's local police department placed a camera within the entrance of the playground. As cars enter the parking lot of the playground, the camera takes a photo of the license plate. While license plate pictures are primarily used to rule out sexual predators at the playground, the pictures can also be used to determine the playground's outreach especially since our IRB wished all surveys to be anonymous. According to license plate data, playground patrons have come from 36 out of 50 states (72%). While the police department is unable to decipher if a car is rented or owned, the data does show that playground patrons do come from a large radius.

Overall Implications

The research presented in this book chapter shows that the universal playground was beneficial for individuals with varying ages and abilities. This finding highlights the need for universally designed playgrounds. Designing playgrounds with playground equipment that is proven effective through rigorous research should be seen as central to community playground builds. Although the social, familial, and cultural benefits of preferred playground equipment may be difficult to quantify, such playgrounds may draw visitors from near and far distances, bringing revenue to the community.

References

ADA Accessibility Guidelines for Play Areas. (2000). Retrieved from http://www.access-board.gov/guidelines-and-standards/buildings-and-sites/about-the-ada-standards/background/ada-accessibility-guidelines-for-play-areas

ADA Standards for Accessible Design. (2010). *2010 ADA Standards for Accessible Design.* Retrieved from https://www.ada.gov/law-and-regs/design-standards/2010-stds/

Boundless Playgrounds. (2010). *Boundless Playgrounds.* Retrieved from http://www.boundlessplaygrounds.org/about/faq.php

Center for Universal Design. (1997). The Principles of Universal Design, Version 2.0.: North Carolina State University.

Crompton, J. L. (2001). The impact of parks on property values: A review of the empirical evidence. *Journal of Leisure Research, 33*(1), 1–31.

Department of Economic and Social Affairs Disability. (2024). *United Nations: Article 19—Living Independently and Being Included in the Community.* Retrieved from https://www.un.org/development/desa/disabilities/convention-on-the-rights-of-persons-with-disabilities/article-19-living-independently-and-being-included-in-the-community.html

Fleiss, J. L. (1981). *Statistical methods for rates and proportions* (2nd ed.). Wiley.

Gibson, J. J. (1950). The theory of affordance. In R. Shaw & J. Bransford (Eds.), *Perceiving, acting, and knowing: Toward an ecological society* (pp. 67–82). Erlbaum.

Levasseur, M., Lussier-Therrien, M., Biron, M. L., Raymond, E., Castonguay, J., Naud, D., Fortier, M., Sevigny, A., Houde, S., & Trembley, L. (2022). Scoping study of definitions of social participation: Update and co-construction of an interdisciplinary consensual definition. *Age and Aging, 51*, 1–13. https://doi.org/10.1093/ageing/afab215

Little, C. E. (1990). *Greenways for America.* John Hopkins University Press.

McConkey, J. (2018). *Inclusive play space design: Transforming communities, fostering social equity.* A presentation at the annual meeting of the National Recreation and Park Association (NRPA), Indianapolis, IN.

Meynhardt, T. (2009). Public value inside: What is public value creation? *International Journal of Public Administration, 3-4*, 192–219. https://doi.org/10.1080/01900690902732632

Moran, M. J., Brookshire, R. A., Coe, D. P., Flynn, J. O., & Shideler, M. J. (2019). Partners through playgrounds: Building a play community. *Children, Youth, and Environments, 29*(1), 153–163. https://doi.org/10.7721/chilyoutenvi.29.1.0153

Sandseter, E. B. H. (2009). Affordances for risky play in preschool: The importance of features in the play environment. *Early Childhood Education. Journal, 36*, 439–446. https://doi:10.1007/s10643-009-0307-2.

Stanton-Chapman, T. L., & Nabors, L. (2024). The influence of a universally designed playground on the play interactions between grandparents and grandchildren. *Children, Youth, and Environments, 34*(2), 84–99. https://doi.org/10.1353/cye.2024.a938206

Stanton-Chapman, T. L., & Rhoades, C. (2018). *The destination playground frequency observation code* [Unpublished manuscript]. University of Cincinnati

Stanton-Chapman, T. L., & Schmidt, E. L. (2016). Special education professionals' perceptions towards accessible playgrounds. *Research and Practice for Persons with Severe Disabilities, 41*(2), 90–100.

Stanton-Chapman, T. L., & Schmidt, E. L. (2017). Creating an inclusive playground for children of all abilities: West Fork Playground in Cincinnati, Ohio. *Children, Youth, and Environments, 27*(3), 124–137. https://doi.org/10.7721/chilyoutenvi.27.3.0124

Stanton-Chapman, T. L., & Schmidt, E. L. (2018). In search of equivalent social participation: What do caregivers of children with disabilities desire regarding inclusive recreational facilities and playgrounds? *Journal of International Special Needs Education, 22*(2), 66–76. https://doi.org/10.9782/16-00035

Stanton-Chapman, T. L., & Schmidt, E. L. (2019). Building playgrounds for children of all abilities: Legal requirements and professional recommendations. *Early Childhood Education Journal, 47*, 509–517. https://doi.org/10.1007/s10643-019-00947-3

Stanton-Chapman, T. L., & Schmidt, E. L. (2021). How do children play? The influence of playground type on children's play styles. *Frontiers in Psychology, 12*, 703–740. https://doi.org/10.3389/fpsyg.2021.703940

Stanton-Chapman, T. L., Schmidt, E. L., Rhoades, C., & Monnin, L. (2020). An observational study of children playing on an inclusive playground and on a universal playground. *International Journal of Social Policy and Education, 2*(2), 37–47. https://doi.org/10.61494/ijspe

Stanton-Chapman, T. L., Rhoades, C., & Schmidt, E. L. (2023). A behavioral investigation of preference for a playground sensory maze. *Journal of Park and Recreation Administration, 41*(2), 100–117. https://doi.org/10.18666/JPRA-2023-10575

Tapp, J. (2021). *Multiple option observation system for experimental studies: MOOSES* [Computer software]. Kennedy Center, Vanderbilt University.

U. S. Architectural & Transportation Barriers Compliance Board. (2004). *Americans with disabilities act and architectural barriers act accessibility guidelines.* Retrieved from https://www.access-board.gov/attachments/article/412/ada-aba.pdf. Provides information on the ADA law and accessibility guidelines.

U. S. Census Bureau. (2019). *American Community Survey Data: 2019.* Retrieved from https://www.census.gov/programs-surveys/acs/about.html

Young, N. A. E. (2021). *Childhood Disability in the United States: 2019.* Retrieved from https://www.census.gov/content/dam/Census/library/publications/2021/acs/acsbr-006.pdf

Chapter 5
Involvement of Young Children with Developmental Disabilities and Chronic Medical Conditions in Extracurricular Activities

Stacy K. Dymond and Alicia R. Pence

Abstract This chapter examines the participation of young children with developmental disabilities and chronic medical conditions in extracurricular activities (ECAs), detailing both benefits and barriers. Despite legal mandates for equal participation, children with disabilities still engage in ECAs at lower rates than their peers, though recent trends show gradual improvement. The chapter synthesizes research on the broad range of ECAs—including sports, clubs, performing arts, and community activities—available in schools and communities, noting significant variability in participation linked to disability type, age, communication needs, and gender. Successful inclusion requires individualized planning, support, and adaptations, such as Individualized Health Plans, natural supports, and accessible environments. Practical strategies for maximizing participation include visual supports, partner/group activities, staff training, and fostering a culture valuing diversity. While highlighting the developmental, social, and health benefits of ECA involvement, the chapter emphasizes persistent challenges for children with extensive support needs and calls for further research and innovative approaches for equitable, meaningful access.

Keywords Children with developmental disabilities · Children with medical conditions · Extracurricular activities · Activity context · Promoting safety; inclusion supports

Extracurricular activities (ECAs) refer to a broad array of organized activities that extend beyond the curriculum provided at school. These activities take place outside

S. K. Dymond (✉)
Special Education, University of Illinois Urbana-Champaign, Champaign, IL, USA
e-mail: sdymond@illinois.edu

A. R. Pence
Special Education, Middle Tennessee State University, Murfreesboro, TN, USA
e-mail: alicia.pence@mtsu.edu

L. Nabors and T. Stanton-Chapman (eds.), *Developmental Disabilities and Chronic Illness in Young Children*, Springer Series on Child and Family Studies,
https://doi.org/10.1007/978-3-032-08523-8_5

Table 5.1 Sample ECAs for young children

School	Community
School clubs	Public library programs
Art/drama	Dance and art classes
Service projects	Girl or Boy Scouts
Choir	4-H
Sports teams	Faith-based activities
Mentoring programs	YMCA programs
Field trips	Summer camps
After school programs	Parks and Recreation offerings

of dedicated class time and do not earn academic credit. Each ECA typically has a particular focus or goal that enables children to explore their interests and develop new skills. The activities involve small to large groups of children with similar interests or skills, and occur on a regular, predictable schedule. Activities are sponsored and/or facilitated by an adult. Some ECAs are open to everyone, some have selection criteria, and some fall somewhere in between. These activities may be free of charge or fee based. A variety of entities offer ECAs including schools, community organizations, and private providers. Examples of common ECAs for young children are described in Table 5.1.

This chapter begins with an overview of existing legislation and research regarding the participation of children with disabilities in ECAs. To date, most research focuses on adolescents; thus, the remainder of the chapter explores applications for young children with disabilities. Specific emphasis is placed on children with extensive support needs (i.e., severe intellectual disability, autism, multiple disabilities) and chronic medical conditions (also known as specialized healthcare needs). A process for selecting appropriate ECAs for this population is described along with strategies for maximizing successful inclusion and active participation. The chapter concludes with implications for research, policy, and practice.

Access to ECAs as Defined by Law

There are three core pieces of legislation that support the inclusion of children with disabilities in ECAs. Each law supports "equal opportunity" of services and programs but varies in the scope of its coverage. The Individuals with Disabilities Education Improvement Act (IDEA, 2004) requires public schools to provide children with disabilities equal opportunity to participate in non-academic activities such as ECAs. Furthermore, schools must ensure that children with disabilities participate in ECAs with peers without disabilities to the maximum extent appropriate and receive supplementary aids and services to support participation. Section 504 of the Rehabilitation Act (1973) applies to public schools but also extends to all organizations that receive federal funding. In 2013, the U.S. Department of Education, Office of Civil Rights issued additional guidance for implementing Section 504 after findings from a U.S. Government Accountability Office (USGAO, 2010) study revealed that students with disabilities participated in school athletic programs at a lower rate than peers without disabilities. This guidance clarifies, but does not change, the requirements of the law. A final piece of legislation that supports the inclusion of children with disabilities in ECAs is the Americans with Disabilities Act (ADA, 1990). Under the ADA (1990), services, programs, and activities offered through state or local government entities, and businesses and non-profits that serve the public, must provide people with disabilities equal opportunity to benefit from their services and programs.

Participation of Children with Disabilities in ECAs

Existing legislation clarifies that children with disabilities must have equal opportunity to participate in ECAs. Despite this legislation, children with disabilities continue to participate in ECAs at significantly lower rates than their peers without disabilities (Cadwallader et al., 2003; Coster et al., 2013; Kim et al., 2024; USGAO, 2010). There is evidence, however, that participation rates are gradually increasing. Findings from the National Longitudinal Transition Study (Liu et al., 2018) show the percentage of children ages 15–18 with an Individualized Education Program (IEP) participating in ECA sports teams and school clubs grew from 61% to 74% between 2003 and 2012. This growth occurred for both school-sponsored and out of school activities, with the greatest growth coming from participation in clubs as opposed to sports.

Research regarding the participation of children with disabilities in ECAs is limited. Much of the research is descriptive in nature and relies on information reported by teachers, parents, and children. In some studies, investigations have encompassed children across a broad range of age groups and disabilities. In other studies, investigations have targeted specific groups of children by age, disability, and/or support needs. Although these variations make it difficult to compare findings across studies and draw conclusions, collectively, the studies provide an emerging picture of how children with disabilities participate in ECAs. Existing research examines five areas. It describes the types of activities in which children with disabilities participate, the context in which activities take place, supports provided to enhance participation, benefits of participation, and barriers that limit participation.

Types of Activities

Children with disabilities participate in a wide range of ECAs related to sports and fitness, clubs, social groups, performing or fine arts, and other special interest groups (Cadwallader et al., 2003; Dymond et al., 2020). Within school-sponsored ECAs, sports are the most frequent ECA in which children with disabilities are reported to participate (Agran et al. 2017; Cadwallader et al., 2003; Dymond et al., 2020). Only one study found children with disabilities participate most frequently in school clubs (Kleinert et al., 2007); these findings may be due to the study's narrower focus on students with moderate and severe intellectual disability (ID). Within community sponsored ECAs, children with disabilities are reported to participate most frequently in religious groups and church social events (Cadwallader et al., 2003; Kleinert et al., 2007). Other activities include scouting, 4-H, youth development groups, recreation activities, lessons, and classes (Agran et al. 2017; Cadwallader et al., 2003; Kleinert et al., 2007).

The types of ECAs in which children participate are dependent, in part, on the activities available in the school and community. Student characteristics such as type of disability, support needs, use of augmentative or alternative communication (AAC), age/grade, and gender also appear related to the types of activities in which children participate. With regard to disability, Lipscomb et al. (2017) found that children ages 13–21 with multiple disabilities and ID were significantly less likely to participate in school clubs or sports than all other children with an IEP. Examining support needs and AAC, Dymond et al. (2020) noted differences in activity participation for children with ID. Children ages 13–21 with severe ID and AAC users were significantly more likely to participate in school clubs and special events than children with mild ID or non-AAC users. Two studies identified differences in type of activity participation between older and younger children. Pappagianopoulos et al. (2024) found that children ages 6–11 with autism spectrum disorder participated more frequently in sports and less frequently in clubs/organizations than children ages 12–17. Kleinert et al. (2007) found that high school students with moderate and severe ID participated significantly more in parks and recreation social activities, school cubs, and choir than elementary age children. With regard to gender, girls with disabilities have lower odds of participating in sport and physical activity compared to boys with and without disabilities and girls without disabilities (Kim et al., 2024).

Activity Context

Most children with disabilities participate in ECAs alongside peers without disabilities (Cadwallader et al., 2003; Dymond et al., 2020). Several organizations also offer activities specifically for children with disabilities (e.g., Special Olympics, Easter Seals, community parks and recreation programs). Existing research indicates that children with extensive support needs participate in disability-oriented ECAs significantly more than children with few support needs. For example, Cadwallader et al. (2003) found that only 5% of children with disabilities ages 13–17 participated in disability-oriented ECAs compared to 18–27% of children with extensive support needs (intellectual/developmental disabilities (ID), multiple disabilities, deaf-blindness, autism, orthopedic disabilities). More recently, Dymond et al. (2020) found that 36% of children with ID ages 13–21 participated in disability-oriented

ECAs. Children with severe ID and AAC users were significantly more likely to participate in disability-oriented ECAs than children with mild ID and/or non-AAC users. Age may also relate to participation. Students ages 19–21 were significantly more likely than middle or high school students to participate in disability-oriented ECAs (Dymond et al., 2020).

Supports

Several researchers have investigated the types of support students with ID receive to enhance their participation in ECAs. One type of support involves teaching students the skills needed to participate in ECAs. For school-age children, this may involve including ECA participation in the IEP (Agran et al., 2020; Pence & Dymond, 2016). Not surprising, most IEP objectives associated with ECA participation target social communication skills. Furthermore, students with severe ID are more likely to work on at least one IEP objective during ECAs than students with mild ID (Agran et al., 2020). A second type of support students may receive to enhance participation is individual assistance during the ECA. A variety of people have successfully supported students during ECAs, including special and general education teachers, paraprofessionals, peers, coaches, club sponsors, and family members (Agran et al., 2020; Kleinert et al. 2007; Pence & Dymond, 2016, 2021). Other types of supports such as assistive technology, AAC, modified instruction, or adapted materials are rarely reported despite their potential for reducing reliance on others for support (Kleinert et al. 2007; Pence & Dymond, 2016). In some instances, children with ID have received few to no supports, with the unspoken expectation that children will "go with the flow" (Pence & Dymond, 2021).

Benefits of Participation

ECAs provide opportunities for children with and without disabilities to explore their interests, learn new skills, and develop friendships outside of the classroom environment. In fact, the development of friendships is one of the most frequently cited benefits of ECA participation for children with disabilities (see Agran et al., 2017; Bills, 2020; Cadwallader et al., 2003; Pappagianopoulos et al., 2024; Pence & Dymond, 2016). Other reported benefits include a sense of acceptance and belonging among peers, increased school engagement and social competence, opportunities to practice functional skills in real contexts, less depression, improved quality of life, and greater self-esteem (Agran et al., 2017; Hoyle et al., 2024; Pappagianopoulos et al., 2024; Pence & Dymond, 2016, 2021; Wachsmuth et al., 2023).

Participation in school sports appears more beneficial for some children with disabilities than participation in school clubs. For students ages 12 and over with mild disabilities, participation in sports (as compared to clubs) reduced the impact of bullying on children's self-esteem, schoolwork, and friendships (Bills, 2020). For children ages 6–17 with autism spectrum disorder, participation in sports (as opposed to clubs) was associated with successful friendships, and for older children (ages 12–17) a decreased likelihood of being diagnosed with depression (Pappagianopoulos et al., 2024).

There is also some evidence to suggest that participation in ECAs has long-term benefits. Children with disabilities who participated in at least one ECA in grade 12 were significantly more likely to complete a postsecondary degree (Palmer et al., 2017). Additionally, childhood participation in group activities is related to better mental health in young adulthood for individuals with developmental disabilities (Hoyle et al., 2024). Although there are a limited number of studies, these studies provide emerging evidence that active engagement in extracurricular activities prior to exiting school may help children develop skills needed for success during early adulthood.

Barriers to Participation

Persistent barriers exist that limit ECA participation by children with disabilities. In some schools and communities, few ECAs exist or the ECAs available do not match the child's interests (Agran et al., 2017; Fisher et al., 2022; Kleinert et al., 2007). Finding appropriate ECAs may be further complicated for children with extensive support needs due to the cognitive, social, and physical demands of many activities (Coster et al., 2013; Kleinert et al., 2007; Pence & Dymond, 2016, 2021). Accommodations and modifications can be made to existing ECAs to support students with extensive support needs; however, some teachers report having insufficient time to plan for their student's participation (Pence & Dymond, 2016) or do not believe it is their responsibility to plan for or monitor students during ECAs (Agran et al., 2017). This challenge is compounded when ECA sponsors lack appropriate skills to support children with disabilities in ways that promote their inclusion and active engagement (Fisher et al., 2022; Pence & Dymond, 2016, 2021; USGAO, 2010). A variety of external factors may also pose barriers to participation. These include parent interest, safety concerns, personnel, equipment, and transportation (Agran et al., 2017; Kleinert et al., 2007; Pence & Dymond, 2016, 2021).

Selecting Appropriate ECAs for Young Children with Extensive Support Needs and Chronic Medical Conditions

Children with disabilities participate in a wide variety of ECAs (Dymond et al., 2020). Although limited research has investigated the participation of young children with extensive support needs and chronic medical conditions, the broader literature provides practical guidance that can be applied when selecting ECAs for this population of children (Ballard & Dymond, 2018; Carter et al., 2010; Pence & Dymond, 2015, 2021; Swedeen et al., 2010). Using the literature, we developed a five-step process for identifying and evaluating potential ECAs. Following these steps will help children, parents, and other educational team members to make informed decisions when selecting ECAs.

Step 1: Examine ECAs Available in the School and Community

One of the most important aspects of including any child in ECAs is knowledge of available opportunities for participation (Pence & Dymond, 2015; Swedeen et al., 2010). Ideally, one would start by searching the school and district website for information. If few details are provided online, contact the child's school and request a list of available ECAs, including clubs, sports teams, and volunteer opportunities. School guidance counselors and administrative staff can be resourceful in providing these details. Activity ideas can also be gained by perusing parent magazines (e.g., *Exceptional Parent*), searching the internet, and contacting local parent groups or organizations (e.g., Down syndrome organization, Autism support group). Consider inquiring about both inclusive and disability-oriented ECAs, as all participation opportunities will come with diverse experiences and potential benefits for the child.

Once school prospects have been fielded, explore the community for additional avenues for participation. Local neighborhood centers (e.g., YMCA, Boys and Girls Club), public libraries, and faith-based organizations are just a few of the opportunities that exist in many communities (see Table 5.1). When searching, it is important to identify free and low-cost options, so that finances will not be a factor in deterring families from participation (Cadwallader et al., 2003). To search for available opportunities, review online community boards such as Facebook groups or the Eventbrite website, as well as offerings found printed in local newspapers, flyers, and bulletins.

Step 2: Assess the Child's Interests

Leisure time can include a range of activities and types of engagement, thus assessing a child's interests begins with understanding how the child enjoys spending their free time. Start by generating a list of three to five questions to ask the child. These questions should be geared toward helping the child think about their own interests, since some young children might not be able to clearly articulate preferences (Carter et al., 2010). Questions related to what the child enjoys doing when feeling well and the characteristics of preferred activities (e.g., active, creative, quiet) will help to determine possible interests and potential new activities to explore.

There are a few strategies that can be used when children are not able to articulate clear preferences. For instance, conducting a preference assessment (Lohrmann-O'Rourke et al., 2000) may help to systematically evaluate various activities and rank the child's interests. Observing the child interacting with toys and other items in the environment may yield additional details about characteristics of preferred activities (e.g., music related, bright colors, soft textures) as well as where and with whom the child enjoys spending leisure time (e.g., with peers, in a group, alone; Pence & Dymond, 2015). Utilizing a short open-ended questionnaire, ask parents and teachers how the child participates within home, school, and community settings. Possible prompts may include inquiries about activities the child naturally gravitates toward, might like to try in the future, or finds challenging but still enjoys.

Step 3: Examine the Family's Interests, Routines, and Concerns

Family interests and routines are important factors to consider when making decisions about including a child with extensive support needs and chronic medical conditions in ECAs. Each family has unique interests that oftentimes stem from familial values and enjoyment in shared experiences. Selecting ECAs that align with family interests may help to ensure that there is ongoing support for the child's involvement (Carter et al., 2010). The family's daily routines are also important to consider since a child's participation in ECAs may alter those routines and place new demands on the family with regard to time, energy, finances, and transportation. Involvement in ECAs that align with the family's interests can be useful for assisting the child to apply skills, used with the family, to other contexts (Carter et al., 2010; Pence & Dymond, 2015). For example, a child whose family enjoys weekly bowling nights, would most likely already have a repertoire of established routines (e.g., preparing to participate, waiting to take turns, rolling the ball during the turn) that could easily be generalized to a community bowling league.

It is important that the family be provided with an opportunity to voice possible apprehensions about participation (Carter et al., 2010; Swedeen et al., 2010). Potential concerns may include how participation in the ECA will impact the child's physical health and safety, accessibility of the activities, availability of appropriate supports, and acceptance by peers (Carter et al., 2010; Swedeen et al., 2010). Concerns should be discussed with the ECA sponsors to ensure that they understand the individualized needs of the child and can adequately address the family's concerns.

Step 4: Compile a List of Potential ECAs

Using the information gathered about available ECAs, make a list of the school and community ECAs that best match the interests of the child and family. This compilation can include inclusive and disability-oriented opportunities that are sponsored by various entities (e.g., school, community organizations, private providers). Rank order the ECAs on the list to clarify those that hold the most promise.

Step 5: Investigate Potential ECAs to Determine Appropriateness

To determine the most ideal ECAs for participation, conduct at least one visit to the top ECAs on the list. During each visit, collect information to determine the skills, abilities, and supports required for participation. Figure 5.1 provides a list of questions that may be useful when assessing various aspects of the ECA. Use the notes section to elaboration on what is observed, identify how the child might participate, and the types of supports the child would need. Jot down questions that arise and speak with the ECA sponsor after the visit to gather more information.

Findings from these visits should guide reflective thinking about the alignment of each ECA with child and family interests. It will be important to also consider how easily the child will be able to adapt or develop new routines to engage in participation. Once the list of options has been narrowed, it may be helpful to have the child explore each opportunity by visiting at least once. After the visit, communicate with the child about how things went. Inquire about what was enjoyed most, what experience was liked least, and if it would be worth returning to the activity again. In some situations, there may be few options that align well with the child's and family's interests. If this situation arises, consider collaborating with others (e.g., teachers, guidance counselors, community organizers) to create a new ECA that matches the child's interests and recruit other students to join (Carter et al., 2010).

Ensuring Successful Inclusion in ECAs

Choosing an ECA that matches the child's and family's interests is only the first step to ensuring a positive experience. The successful inclusion of young children with disabilities in ECAs requires purposeful planning, careful monitoring, ongoing evaluation, and occasional adjustments. Perhaps most important is the planning that occurs prior to the first day of ECA participation. For children with extensive support needs (i.e., severe intellectual disability, autism, multiple disabilities), ECA sponsors and parents need to consider how to structure the environment to promote meaningful inclusion and active engagement in activities. Additionally, when children have

Extracurricular Activity (ECA) Questions	Yes/No
Environmental Considerations	
1. Is the setting physically accessible?	
2. Does the ECA appear to be welcoming for all children?	
3. Is the environment structured to promote partner and small group activities?	
4. Are children appropriately supervised?	
5. Are there any safety concerns?	
6. Is the environment appropriate for the child (e.g., lighting, smells, sounds, temperature)?	
Child Engagement	
7. Can the child actively participate in the core ECA activities with or without assistance?	
8. Is remote participation allowed if needed?	
9. Are individualized supports/accommodations available to help maximize participation?	
10. Can a child participate at their own pace, and take breaks as needed?	
Individualized Supports	
11. Are ECA sponsors trained to work with children with chronic medical conditions, especially in the case of an emergency?	
12. Do ECA sponsors know how to use a variety of communication modes, like AAC and visual/picture schedules?	
13. Can parents or family members be present during activities to support the child?	
14. Are peers utilized as partners/buddies?	
15. Are peers trained to provide individualized supports?	
Other Considerations	
16. Is specialized equipment available (e.g., adaptive bowling ramps, modified art supplies)?	
17. Are there clear routines that the child can learn to follow?	
18. Is transportation readily available?	
19. Is the ECA sponsor open to working together to create a plan for supporting the child?	

Fig. 5.1 Checklist for evaluating and selecting ECAs for young children with disabilities and chronic medical conditions

chronic medical conditions, procedures must be in place to ensure the child's safety and accommodate healthcare needs during activities. Although ECAs for young children focus on fun and enjoyment, certain conditions, when present, will ensure those with extensive support needs and chronic medical conditions maximally benefit from their ECA experiences.

Promoting Health and Safety

Parents and teachers have voiced concern about the safety of children with disabilities and chronic medical conditions, particularly when they are participating in activities with peers without disabilities (Ballard & Dymond, 2018, 2023; Carter et al., 2010; Pence & Dymond, 2021; Swedeen et al., 2010). These concerns may prevent children from accessing ECAs if not appropriately addressed. Safety is certainly a concern for all children, regardless of disability, so clarifying existing safety procedures within an ECA is important. There are several additional steps that can be taken to protect the health and wellness of children with chronic medical conditions. These steps will help to alleviate potential concerns that may exist among parents, ECA sponsors, and participants.

Prior to a child with chronic medical conditions entering an ECA, it is paramount that all staff associated with the ECA are knowledgeable about the child's medical condition and the supports the child requires during the ECA. How this information is shared depends on the child's unique needs. One option is to share the child's individual health plan (IHP) with ECA sponsors. All school-age children with chronic medical conditions should have an IHP that is developed by the child's parents, the child, and the child's healthcare providers (i.e., physician, school nurse). The purpose of the IHP is to clarify the child's nursing needs while at school so that consistent health care is provided across settings (National Association of School Nurses, 2020). Types of information communicated in an IHP may include such topics as medication administration, environmental concerns (e.g., allergens, lighting), healthcare procedures, transportation requirements, and emergency procedures. An IHP also specifies staff responsibilities and required training, and how the child will participate in their own health care.

The school nurse oversees the development and implementation of the IHP at school, thus when children who have IHPs are considering participation in school-sponsored ECAs, it is important to inform the school nurse. The nurse will work with the educational team, including the parent and ECA sponsor, to determine how the child's healthcare needs can be addressed during the ECA and provide training to the sponsor if needed. For activities that are not school sponsored, it is important for parents to communicate their child's healthcare needs with the sponsoring organization. If the organization does not have a written form for documenting healthcare needs, the parent may wish to share selected sections of the child's IHP with the sponsor to begin discussion about how health and safety for their child will be maintained. Alternatively, if a child does not have an IHP, sample forms are widely available on the Internet and can be downloaded and used when discussing the child's support needs with the sponsor. Community organizations that provide ECAs are not required to provide nursing services listed in the IHP, therefore it may be necessary for parents to identify additional supports to ensure their child's safety when participating.

Structuring the Environment

The ECA sponsor(s) plays a critical role in structuring the environment to promote each child's meaningful inclusion and active engagement. Despite the importance of their role, many sponsors have limited experience working with children with extensive support needs and may struggle to understand how to include them in the ECA (Fisher et al., 2022; Pence & Dymond, 2016, 2021; USGAO, 2010). Lack of knowledge, training, and experience can result in feelings of frustration and anxiety among ECA sponsors, leading to children being inadvertently excluded from activities due to insufficient support or supervision (Pence & Dymond, 2021). To avoid this situation, members of the child's educational team can assist sponsors to plan for the child's inclusion and offer intermittent training and support to the sponsor, child, and other ECA participants. Intermittent training might include demonstrating techniques for working with the child (e.g., positioning, prompting, communication), sharing tips on how to promote interactions between peers with and without disabilities, or providing guidance on how to handle physical or emotional changes the child is experiencing due to taking a new medication.

Planning for a child's inclusion begins with examining the activities that occur during the ECA. These activities can be divided into core routines that happen every day and intermittent activities that are variable or happen less frequently. For example, routines within an after-school arts program might include arrival, getting out materials, creating a project, clean up, and departure. Intermittent activities might include variations in the types of art projects created and the inclusion of occasional special events such as a guest artist who works with the children or an art show for families showcasing the children's work. Each of these routines can be analyzed to determine how peers without disabilities typically participate followed by discussing how the child with extensive support needs will participate. This process of analyzing activities is referred to as an ecological inventory (Pence & Dymond, 2015). Using this process may also help to identify IEP objectives the child could practice during the ECA and new skills that could be targeted for instruction (e.g., social and communication skills). The child's teacher and parents can facilitate skill development by teaching the skills at home and at school and showing the ECA sponsor how to teach the same skills during the ECA.

The type and amount of support a child might need within the ECA setting depends on the nature of the activities. Identifying the correct amount of support can be difficult. Too little support may limit a child's inclusion in activities and too much support may interfere with access to peers and the development of friendships (Pence & Dymond, 2021). Supplementary aids and services specified in the IEP (e.g., AAC device, specialized equipment, frequent breaks, staff support) provide direction regarding the types of supports a child may need. These supports should be considered when mapping out which, if any, supports will be provided during each activity that occurs within the ECA. Some activities may not require added supports beyond what is normally provided for all children.

One of the most common types of supports provided to children with extensive support needs is a one-on-one adult assistant. There are many ways to structure the environment to reduce the need for an additional adult by creating opportunities for natural supports (Carter et al., 2010). Natural supports refer to the supports that are already available in the setting, such as the ECA sponsor, peers, and volunteers. The ECA sponsor can promote natural supports by structuring the environment to have children work in pairs or small groups and teaching them to support each other. A child with extensive support needs benefits from seeing peers model various skills (e.g., communication, social, task related) and peers are more likely to interact with the child if he or she is not seated next to an adult (Giangreco, 2010). Additionally, these grouping arrangements can facilitate the child's partial participation in activities. With partial participation (Ferguson & Baumgart, 1991) a child completes the parts of a task that they can complete independently and someone else completes the other parts or assists the child to complete the other parts. For example, a child who has difficulty squeezing a glue bottle may have a peer apply the glue while the child completes the rest of the art project. Alternatively, the ECA sponsor may assist the child to squeeze the bottle by providing hand-over-hand assistance if the child lacks the strength to do so himself.

There are many strategies, beyond those previously mentioned, for structuring the environment to promote meaningful inclusion and active engagement (see Table 5.2). Educational teams play an important role in collaborating with ECA sponsors to plan for a child's inclusion, but they also are instrumental in helping sponsors acquire the skills needed to successfully support children. Some ECA sponsors may benefit from additional coaching to implement the practices in Table 5.2. Checking in regularly with the sponsor may help identify challenges and work through solutions. For sponsors with limited experience, adding a co-sponsor from the educational team may provide support for co-planning events and opportunities to model techniques for structuring the environment. This support can be faded over time as the sponsor becomes more comfortable with their role.

Implications for Research, Policy, and Practice

Children with and without disabilities benefit from participation in ECAs (e.g., Pappagianopoulos et al., 2024; Philippe et al., 2022). Existing research suggests that despite the benefits, barriers continue to exist that prevent children from accessing ECAs. Furthermore, children with the most extensive support needs participate in ECAs at lower rates than children with fewer support needs. Additional research is needed to explore how children with extensive support needs are successfully included in ECAs with peers without disabilities and strategies that facilitate their active engagement. Future research might also investigate the participation of young children and children with chronic medical conditions in ECAs to determine supports that facilitate their participation.

Table 5.2 Structuring the ECA Environment for Young Children with Disabilities and Chronic Medical Conditions

Ideas for structuring the ECA environment
Activities
Determine how children will participate or partially participate in each activity
Embed opportunities for children with disabilities to work on priority IEP objectives
Clarify when and where health related supports will be provided
Establish roles and responsibilities for each adult (e.g., ECAExtracurricular activities sponsor, volunteers, 1:1 assistant)
Supports
Provide supplementary aids and services identified in the IEP
Clarify who will provide health related supports including the child's role
Use natural supports whenever possible (e.g., ECA sponsor, participants, volunteers)
Group children for activities (partners, small groups, rotating groups) and/or assign roles
Enlist peers in problem solving how to include a child in an activity
Identify peer buddies for specific activities (e.g., clean up)
Use visuals, social stories, and other accommodations to facilitate understanding
Setting
Arrange the environment to promote physical accessibility
Identify where healthcare documents and equipment will be safely stored
Adjust lighting and sound levels if needed
Post rules and behavioral expectations
Identify and address potential safety concerns
Training
Provide training and intermittent support for ECA sponsors
Ensure time for the ECA sponsor and education team to plan, evaluate, and adjust activities
Provide peers with information and strategies to support children with extensive support needs
Teach children skills at home and in school that are needed to increase participation in the ECA
Culture
Create a culture that everyone belongs
Teach children respect for individual differences
Recognize that everyone can help someone, and everyone can benefit from help
Reinforce collaboration
Engage children in developing rules and expectations for behavior

Note. Educational teams may find it useful to develop a written plan that documents specific strategies that will be used to structure the environment (e.g., types of supports provided, room arrangement). This plan can be revisited periodically and adjusted as appropriate

Current legislation (i.e., IDEA, Section 504, ADA) fully supports the participation of children with disabilities in ECAs. As evidenced by the guidance issued in 2013 for implementing Section 504 by the U.S. Department of Education, Office of Civil Rights, there may not be uniform clarity regarding how to include children with disabilities in ECAs. Whether additional federal guidance is needed to fully implement current laws is dependent, in part, on whether the rate of participation by children with disabilities continues to significantly lag behind children without disabilities (Cadwallader et al., 2003; Coster et al., 2013; Kim et al., 2024; USGAO, 2010). Schools and community organizations may find it helpful to clarify their policies for including children with disabilities in ECAs, examine rates of participation of children with and without disabilities, and determine whether changes are needed to foster greater inclusion of children with disabilities.

Despite limited research specifically focused on ECAs for young children with chronic medical conditions, there are several key implications for practice that can be drawn from the existing literature and current legislation. First, schools and community organizations must provide equal opportunity for children with disabilities to access ECAs. Second, child and family interests should drive the selection of ECAs, and family concerns must be addressed. Third, potential ECA matches should be evaluated by visiting the ECA and talking with the ECA sponsor. Fourth, once an ECA is selected, procedures must be in place to ensure the child's safety and accommodate healthcare needs during activities. Lastly, collaborative planning that involves the educational team and ECA sponsor will enable the ECA setting to be structured in a manner that promotes meaningful inclusion and active engagement for children with extensive support needs.

References

Agran, M., Achola, E., Nixon, C. A., Wojcik, A., Cain, I., Thoma, C., et al. (2017). Participation of students with intellectual and developmental disabilities in extracurricular activities: Does inclusion end at 3:00? *Education and Training in Autism and Developmental Disabilities, 52*(1), 3–12.

Agran, M., Dymond, S., Rooney-Kron, M., & Martin, J. (2020). Examining whether student participation in school-sponsored extracurricular activities is represented in IEPs. *Intellectual and Developmental Disabilities, 58*(6), 472–485. https://doi.org/10.1352/1934-9556-58.6.472

Americans with Disabilities Act (ADA) of 1990, 42 U.S.C. §12101 *et seq.* (1990).

Ballard, S. L., & Dymond, S. K. (2018). Inclusive education for secondary-age students with severe disabilities and complex health care needs. *Intellectual and Developmental Disabilities, 56*(6), 427–441. https://doi.org/10.1352/1934-9556-56.6.427

Ballard, S., & Dymond, S. K. (2023). Beliefs about secondary-age students with extensive support needs participating in their health care at school. *Research and Practice for Persons with Severe Disabilities, 48*(2), 92–107. https://doi.org/10.1177/15407969231173932

Bills, K. L. (2020). Helping children with disabilities combat negative socio-emotional outcomes caused by bullying through extracurricular activities. *Journal of Human Behavior in the Social Environment, 30*(5), 573–585. https://doi.org/10.1080/10911359.2020.1718052

Cadwallader, T. W., Wagner, M., & Garza, N. (2003). Participation in extracurricular activities. In M. Wagner, T. W. Cadwallader, C. Marder, R. Cameto, D. Cardoso, N. Garza, et al. (Eds.),

Life outside the classroom for youth with disabilities. A report from the National Longitudinal Transition Study-2 (NLTS2) (pp. 4-2–4-8). SRI International.
Carter, E. W., Swedeen, B., Moss, C. K., & Pesko, M. J. (2010). "What are you doing after school?": Promoting extracurricular involvement for transition-age youth with disabilities. *Intervention in School and Clinic, 45*(5), 275–283.
Coster, W., Law, M., Bedell, G., Liljenquist, K., Kao, Y. C., Khetani, M., & Teplicky, R. (2013). School participation, supports and barriers of students with and without disabilities. *Child: Care, Health and Development, 39*(4), 535–543. https://doi.org/10.1111/cch.12046
Dymond, S. K., Rooney, M. A., Burke, M., & Agran, M. (2020). Characteristics of secondary age students with intellectual disability who participate in school sponsored extracurricular activities. *Journal of Special Education, 54*(1), 51–62. https://doi.org/10.1177/002246691985 1194
Ferguson, D. L., & Baumgart, D. (1991). Partial participation revisited. *Journal of the Association for Persons with Severe Handicaps, 16*(4), 218–227.
Fisher, K. M., Shannon-Baker, P., Greer, K., & Serianni, B. (2022). Perspectives of students with disabilities and their parents on influences and barriers to joining and staying in extracurricular STEM activities. *The Journal of Special Education, 56*(2), 110–120. https://doi.org/10.1177/00224669211 0541
Giangreco, M. F. (2010). One-to-one paraprofessionals for students with disabilities in inclusive classrooms: Is conventional wisdom wrong? *Intellectual and Developmental Disabilities, 48*(1), 1–13. https://doi.org/10.1352/1934-9556-48.1.1
Hoyle, J. N., Warren-Findlow, J., Wallace, L., Laditka, J. N., & Laditka, S. B. (2024). Time in childhood extracurricular activity and mental health of young adults with developmental disability. *Disability and Health Journal, 17*(4), 101671. https://doi.org/10.1016/j.dhjo.2024.101671
Individuals with Disabilities Education Improvement Act, 20 U.S.C. § 1400 (2004).
Kim, M., Jung, J., & Yun, J. (2024). Prevalence of school-based extracurricular sport and physical activity participation among children with disabilities. *International Journal of Disability, Development and Education, 71*(1), 1–12. https://doi.org/10.1080/1034912X.2022.2060947
Kleinert, H. L., Miracle, S., & Sheppard-Jones, K. (2007). Including students with moderate and severe intellectual disabilities in school extracurricular and community recreation activities. *Intellectual and Developmental Disabilities, 45*(1), 46–55.
Lipscomb, S., Haimson, J., Liu, A. Y., Burghardt, J., Johnson, D. R., & Thurlow, M. L. (2017). Preparing for life after high school: The characteristics and experiences of youth in special education. *Findings from the National Longitudinal Transition Study 2012. Volume 2: Comparisons across disability groups: Executive summary* (NCEE 2017-4019). U.S. Department of Education, Institute of Education Sciences, National Center for Education Evaluation and Regional Assistance.
Liu, A. Y., Lacoe, J., Lipscomb, S., Haimson, J., Johnson, D. R., & Thurlow, M. L. (2018). Preparing for life after high school: The characteristics and experiences of youth in special education. Findings from the National Longitudinal Transition Study 2012. *Volume 3: Comparisons over time (Full report)* (NCEE 2018-4007). U.S. Department of Education, Institute of Education Sciences, National Center for Education Evaluation and Regional Assistance.
Lohrmann-O'Rourke, S., Browder, D. M., & Brown, F. (2000). Guidelines for conducting socially valid systematic preference assessments. *Journal of the Association for Persons with Severe Handicaps, 25*(1), 42–53. https://doi.org/10.2511/rpsd.25.1.42
National Association of School Nurses. (2020). *Use of individualized healthcare plans to support school health services (Position Statement).* Author. https://www.nasn.org/nasn-resources/professional-practice-documents/position-statements/ps-ihps
Palmer, A. N., Elliott, W., & Cheatham, G. A. (2017). Effects of extracurricular activities on postsecondary completion for students with disabilities. *The Journal of Educational Research, 110*(2), 151–158. https://doi.org/10.1080/00220671.2015.1058221
Pappagianopoulos, J., Rouch, E., & Mazurek, M. O. (2024). Extracurricular activity participation among autistic children and adolescents: Buffer for internalizing conditions and foundation for

friendship? *Journal of Autism and Developmental Disorders, 54*, 4444–4455. https://doi.org/10.1007/s10803-023-06158-5

Pence, A. R., & Dymond, S. K. (2015). Extracurricular school clubs: A time for fun and learning. *Teaching Exceptional Children, 47*(5), 281–288. https://doi.org/10.1177/0040059915580029

Pence, A. R., & Dymond, S. K. (2016). Teachers' beliefs about the participation of students with severe disabilities in school clubs. *Research and Practice for Persons with Severe Disabilities, 41*(1), 52–68. https://doi.org/10.1177/1540796915626009

Pence, A. R., & Dymond, S. K. (2021). The participation of secondary students with severe disabilities in school clubs. *Intellectual and Developmental Disabilities, 59*(4), 335–351. https://doi.org/10.1352/1934-9556-59.4.335

Philippe, F. L., Gingras, M. P., Ghassemi-Bakhtiari, N., Poulin, F., Robitaille, J., Denault, A. S., et al. (2022). Organized civic and non-civic activities as predictors of academic GPA in high school students. *Applied Developmental Science, 27*(2), 189–204. https://doi.org/10.1080/10888691.2022.2053127

Section 504 of the Rehabilitation Act of 1973, 29 U.S.C § 794 (1973).

Swedeen, B. L., Carter, E. W., & Molfenter, N. (2010). Getting everyone involved: Identifying transition opportunities for youth with severe disabilities. *Teaching Exceptional Children, 43*(2), 38–49.

United States Government Accountability Office. (2010). *Students with disabilities: More information and guidance could improve opportunities in physical education and athletics* (GAO-10-519). Author.

Wachsmuth, S. T., Lewis, T. J., & Gage, N. A. (2023). Exploring extracurricular activity participation, school engagement, and social competence for students with emotional and behavioral disorders. *Behavioral Disorders, 48*(4), 255–268. https://doi.org/10.1177/01987429231166675

Chapter 6
Siblings of Disabled Children

Nikki Donnelly and Heather Dee Frankovich

Abstract This chapter explores the experiences of siblings of children with disabilities through Family Systems Theory, emphasizing that a child's disability affects every family member's roles, emotions, and connections. It examines both challenges—feelings of invisibility ("glass child" phenomenon), resentment, guilt, isolation, and parentification—and opportunities for growth in empathy, maturity, and pride. The chapter highlights how sibling age, gender, family communication, and the child's independence influence sibling relationships and well-being. Scenarios and personal accounts show how siblings may feel neglected or burdened by responsibility when their own needs are overlooked. Strategies and interventions include dedicated time, open communication, peer and therapeutic support, role clarification, and acknowledgment of feelings. The chapter calls for intentional support for siblings, offering recommendations to promote resilience, well-being, and positive relationships within families affected by disability.

Keywords Siblings of children with disabilities · Feelings of siblings · Supporting siblings · Programs for siblings

Introduction

Siblings play an important role in the families of children with disabilities. Given that siblings share the longest relationships in life, they can have the most impact on each other. This is true for sibling relationships in general and likely even more so for siblings where one or more experiences a disability. One would expect the typical sibling experiences of joy, rivalry, support, and shared experiences, but one should also consider the unique experiences of the sibling of a child with a disability and that impact on that sibling.

N. Donnelly (✉) · H. D. Frankovich
Sibling Leadership Network, National Headquarters, Chicago, IL, USA
e-mail: nikki.donnelly@oregonsibs.org

L. Nabors and T. Stanton-Chapman (eds.), *Developmental Disabilities and Chronic Illness in Young Children*, Springer Series on Child and Family Studies,
https://doi.org/10.1007/978-3-032-08523-8_6

Using a Family Systems Theory view, the family unit is an interconnected, interdependent emotional unit where each member's behaviors, emotions, and roles impact and are impacted by the others within the unit (Bowen, 1966). Thus, having an individual within the unit that experiences a disability will impact all others within the unit. This impact can vary based upon the gender, closeness in age, and support needs of the child with a disability (Heller & Arnold, 2010). Many siblings report feeling like the "glass child" (TedX Talks, 2010) where they feel invisible and in the shadows (Knecht et al., 2014). Feelings of responsibility, jealousy, resentment, or guilt may be present; however, so might feelings of pride and empathy, as well as increased maturity. In this chapter, we will discuss how siblings of an individual with a disability are impacted, both the challenges and positive aspects, and provide insight into the support needs for these siblings as well as recommendations for families, professionals, and researchers. The authors use quotes to illustrate key points, and these quotes are paraphrased from experiences with clients, parents, and children.

Role of the Sibling in the Family

When one sibling has a disability, there is likely increased contact as compared to traditional siblings (Carr, 2005). Siblings will often be involved in therapies, attending appointments, and providing care support. The role and the relationship between siblings are impacted by the age and gender of the sibling, as well as the nature of the brother or sister's disability (Carr, 2005; Hodapp & Urbano, 2007; Jajodia & Roy, 2023). In a study by Hodapp and Urbano (2007), siblings of a brother/sister with Down Syndrome reported less depression and better health than siblings of someone with autism. However, Orsmond and Seltzer (2000) highlight that siblings of adults with autism report more of a positive impact on their relationships with their parents than siblings of adults with Down Syndrome. Additionally, for brothers, relationships with their siblings of the same gender were stronger than those of the opposite gender (Orsmond & Seltzer, 2000). Finally, when challenging behaviors are present, siblings tend to take on less of a caregiving role (Saxena, 2015).

Other factors that impact the relationship between siblings include the level of independence of the sibling with a disability and the degree of effective communication within the family (Paul et al., 2022). Siblings are more likely to express joy when they experience shared positive interactions with their brother or sisters with a disability (Rixon et al., 2025). They share decreased negative perspectives regarding the future when their brother or sister with a disability live outside of the parental home (Calio & Higgins-D'Alessandro, 2021; Seltzer et al., 2001).

Open communication between parents and siblings regarding future caregiving roles may enhance the relationship between the sibling and brother/sister with a disability (Marks et al., 2005). Siblings often report feeling that they take on more responsibilities than their peers and that the expectation of involvement with their brother or sister parallels parental involvement such as isolation, guilt, concerns regarding the future, and guilt (Calio & Higgins-D'Alessandro, 2021; Lobato et al.,

2011; Neece et al., 2010; Jajodia & Roy, 2023; Rodger & Tooth, 2004). Families with more involved siblings have been identified as being more cohesive, holding stronger values of independence for the child with a disability and have higher levels of family organization (Benson & Karlof, 2008; Taylor et al., 2023). Open communication, where the sibling feels their needs and desires are heard and valued, can decrease their feelings of invisibility and creates a space where they feel they can are understood and relates to increased sibling satisfaction with future planning (Benson & Karlof, 2008; Marks et al., 2005; Orm et al., 2022; Taylor et al., 2023).

The relationship of siblings to their brothers or sisters with a disability often center around a support role within their family. This can look similar to a typical sibling role such as an older sibling gathering diapering supplies with their parents, to a unique role such as participating in and supporting the speech therapy of their brother or sister with autism. As parents age the siblings may take on more of a direct caretaker or care management role for their sibling with a disability (Hayden et al., 2023; Marquis et al., 2019; Saxena & Adamsons, 2013). For example, some siblings may co-reside and be full-time caregivers for their brother or sister; whereas some siblings may live out of state and monitor the care to ensure quality of care or to not have any involvement at all. Typically, female siblings are more likely to take on the caregiving role and provide emotional support for their brother/sister with a disability (Saxena, 2015). Older siblings also tend to take on this role as well (Casale et al., 2021).

Impacts on Sibling

Many siblings have shared the positive impact that having a brother or sister with a disability has had on their lives. Siblings have disclosed an increased sense of personal well-being, such as functioning well, having good health and high levels of reward from being a sibling (Heller & Arnold, 2010; Paul et al., 2022). The closer the sibling feels to their brother or sister, emotionally, the more likely they are to report feelings of well-being (Heller & Arnold, 2010). Siblings can feel a sense of pride in viewing their brother or sister with a disability as "normal" (Calio & Higgins-D'Alessandro, 2021; McGraw & Walker, 2007) and recognize their opportunity for enhanced morality (McGraw & Walker, 2007).

Siblings tend to have more positive self-esteem as well as increased maturity and empathy (Kaminsky & Dewey, 2002; Taylor et al., 2023). Siblings may become the over-achiever as they feel pressure to be perfect to "make up" for their disabled brother or sister, or to ensure they are not putting additional stress on the household for having their own challenges (Hanvey et al., 2022). It is, however, important to note that too much empathy and maturity can also be considered a challenge in that the person may show signs of co-dependency and/or parentification. Healthy levels of maturity can facilitate independence and self-esteem for young children and adults. In healthy amounts, increased empathy can manifest in identifying and engaging with those that society may have marginalized. In fact, most siblings tend to go into humanities professions (Calio & Higgins-D'Alessandro, 2021; Marks et al., 2005; Saxena, 2015) such as becoming special education teachers, mental health professionals, or lawyers. Many siblings become advocates for their siblings, whether it be in advocating for their individual needs for services, etc. or for the disability community through local, state, or national policy change (Lee et al., 2024). These positive aspects for the sibling can manifest in resiliency and in having a sense of pride for themselves and their brother or sister with a disability.

Some positive sibling traits, when taken to an unhealthy level, can be a cause for concern. Feelings of responsibility may take on both a positive and a negative effect for the individual. For example, young children may handle responsibilities such as assisting with in-home medical procedures. This allows them to feel a sense of contribution to the family and to their siblings with a disability. However, a too increased sense of responsibility can have negative impacts. These impacts may vary across the lifespan of the sibling. For example, a teen preparing to graduate from high school may forgo leaving for college due to their feeling they need to stay to emotionally support their parents with the impact of their sister's behavioral episodes. An adult sibling may have difficulty holding a fulfilling career due to the need to take time off work to support the needs of their sister with complex medical issues. Parentification and loyalty binds can occur anytime throughout the lifetime of the sibling that has unhealthy feelings of responsibility and thus should be a topic of discussion within families (Hanvey et al., 2022; Hooper, 2007; Stoneman, 2005; Tomeny et al., 2017).

Sibling Challenges

Challenges surrounding internalized behaviors and externalized behaviors have been identified for siblings, with there being more evidence of internalized behaviors than externalized behaviors (Hanvey et al., 2022; Rossiter & Sharpe, 2001). Emotional experiences such as grief, lack of parental availability and time, separation anxiety, feelings of rejection and/or feeling unimportant, ignored or neglected as well as general sadness, anxiety and shame may be present (Hanvey et al., 2022; Knecht et al., 2014). Siblings have also reported a higher level of unmet emotional needs which impacts their well-being. (Hanvey et al., 2022) Although these may be difficult topics for families to discuss, doing so while providing a space for open and honest communication, will affect the impact of these feelings on the sibling. This open communication is critical given the higher rates of treatment for depression (Liu et al., 2011; Marquis et al., 2019) in siblings, as well as somatic complaints such as headaches or stomach aches (Liu et al., 2011) In fact, a lack of social support from others with shared experiences has been shown to contribute to siblings' feeling of social isolation, stress, and other negative mental health conditions (Bellin & Kovacs, 2006; Hanvey et al., 2022; Simich et al., 2003).

Internalized Behaviors

Emotional challenges experienced by siblings may include internalized feelings of resentment, guilt, anger, and/or isolation (Brinkman et al., 2023; Calio & Higgins-D'Alessandro, 2021; Hanvey et al., 2022; Kovacs et al., 2019). These internalizing behaviors are likely due to the disparity of attention reportedly received by siblings from many of the adults in their lives (Hanvey et al., 2022).

Resentment Resentment is an internalized feeling that siblings may experience. Sibling involvement with their brother or sister with a disability often parallel those of parents (Calio & Higgins-D'Alessandro, 2021). Young children, with little to no experiences outside of their family unit, may view this level of involvement as typical and experience resentment as they enter adulthood and reflect on their youth. For young children, their resentment may be better aligned to lack of parental attention; whereas a child with a disability may be the focus of the family and utilize more of the family's emotional and financial resources, leaving the sibling to potentially receive less attention from parents, extended family, and friends (Hanvey et al., 2022; Knecht et al., 2014). Siblings have reported that due to the nature of the sibling needs and time demands, they often felt unseen, and their needs were not recognized. These feelings resulted in significant levels of frustration and sadness (Hanvey et al., 2022).

Another cause of resentment arises when there is a mismatch of expectations among the disabled and non-disabled children. Siblings often report feeling they carry excessive responsibilities, that their brother or sister is favored in the family, or that their brothers or sisters are overprotected or permitted to behave in ways that they are not allowed (Rixon et al., 2025; Saxena & Adamsons, 2013). However, as the child grows older and begins to realize the uniqueness of their family, they may begin to show resentment for the role they had to play in the family. Older siblings may have resentment toward their parents for their responsibility to take on a caregiving/care management role (Hanvey et al., 2022). A lack of future planning and/or a lack of including the sibling in the planning process may also be a cause of resentment (Calio & Higgins-D'Alessandro, 2021; Saxena, 2015).

Supporting siblings through the emotions that bring up feelings of resentment can be done through efforts such as setting aside an evening a month or a full day a year to connect with the sibling as an individual. This allows for time to connect and learn about their personal desires and for them to express their feelings through open communication (Hanvey et al., 2022).

It never ends. Every time there is a crisis with my sib, my parents call me and expect me to fix, solve, direct, or handle it for them. Yesterday, they called me ten times at the office, putting my job in jeopardy. That evening, I had to work on a resource list and continue to field calls, this time from my mom, who was so emotionally distraught by this episode where my brother had left the living room destroyed. I only got 4 hours of sleep. After I handled it all, I had not a single thank you. In fact, I don't expect another call from my parents until there is another crisis. I do not exist unless I am needed to fix something.

Guilt Siblings may also feel guilt for a variety of reasons. First, conflicting emotions such as experiencing embarrassment at the same time as feeling love and loyalty to their brother or sister may occur (Hanvey et al., 2022; Kovacs et al., 2019). Disagreements and negative thoughts such as anger (Calio & Higgins-D'Alessandro, 2021; Hanvey et al., 2022; Kovacs et al., 2019) toward the other, which are typical in all sibling relationships, can cause siblings to feel guilt for their thoughts and actions as they take the perspective of being unsympathetic or unkind to their sibling with a disability.

Younger siblings may experience guilt for developmentally surpassing their brother or sister, or for participating in life milestones that their sibling with a disability may not have the opportunity or ability to do (Kovacs et al., 2019, Rochefort et al., 2023). These feelings may surface throughout a lifetime during events such as going to a school dance or a school football game with friends, driving a car, moving out of the family home, getting married, having children, etc. Younger siblings may also feel responsibility for causing the disability such as if they were being punished for something that they said or did (Saxena & Adamsons, 2013).

Adult siblings may feel guilty for moving away from home (Hanvey et al., 2022) and for not being able to offer constant support to their brother or sister as they begin to live independent lives (Hanvey et al., 2022). They may view the ease of their own life when compared to their brother or sister and experience guilt around their own health and abilities (Hanvey et al., 2022).

Supporting siblings through feelings of guilt may be best addressed through peer and group support to build a social network of others with shared experiences where authentic expressions can be shared. Additionally, for young children who deal with embarrassment, a simple script for them to use when peers ask them questions about their brother or sister may be helpful. Practicing how to handle questions and uncomfortable situations can empower them to act and decrease feelings of embarrassment. Finally, whether through open communication, support groups, or therapeutic interventions, helping siblings understand that conflicting emotions such as love, and embarrassment, are normal and that they do not need to feel guilt for having those feelings. Therapeutic interventions can also support parents to be active listeners with a non-judgmental presence. Providing a non-judgmental presence and active listening through the use of reflective responses and without the need to "fix" things, can aid in the validation of the sibling's unique experience.

I am about to get married. In a typical family, it would be pretty standard to have your sister as the maid of honor. I feel so terrible, but I do not want my sister in my wedding party. I love her, but my whole life it's always been about her. I just want one day—ONE DAY- where I get to be seen and not pushed into the shadows of my sister and her disability. I know that I will be judged and told I am selfish if I do this. It will be super hurtful to my sis if I don't have her in the wedding party. So, as usual, I'll do "what I am supposed to do" for everyone else so that they are happy. I already feel guilty for falling in love and getting married, when my sister probably never will get to. I can't win.

I was invited to a trampoline birthday party and my sib was not because he has CP and is in a wheelchair. I feel so bad that I can have friends and do things while he is left out. Sometimes, it makes it hard for me to even have fun because I feel guilty leaving him behind.

Anger Siblings can experience feelings of anger for a variety of reasons. First, and tied to jealousy and resentment, siblings may be angry at the parents or their sibling with a disability for taking many of the family's physical and emotional resources, such as parental time and attention. Siblings may displace anger about a sibling's disability and its impact in their lives onto the parent, a safer target. The parent becomes the outlet for these emotions because of the perceived emotional safety, strength, and authority compared to their brother or sister with a disability (Burbidge & Minnes, 2014; Giallo et al., 2012). Anger may also manifest due to social impacts such as attending the same school and hearing peers say unkind things about their sibling with a disability. This anger may be directed toward the brother or sister with the disability for not "behaving" at school and/or at the peers who say unkind words. Into adulthood, siblings may become angry at the lack of or insufficient support afforded to their brother or sister with a disability. They may experience anger and resentment for having to take on a care management role if their parents do not advocate for the needs of their sibling with a disability or have become unable to do so.

Supporting siblings through feelings of anger may be best done through active listening and providing a safe, non-judgmental space for a young child or adult to express their feelings. This space may be filled by the parent, close family friend, or community resources. For younger siblings, therapeutic interventions such as play therapy can provide safe expression of painful feelings. Having a safe space to release these feelings when they arise can support the sibling in expressing their feelings of anger in a healthy manner.

I am an adult with my own family and have a brother with severe autism. He struggles with emotional regulation and is prone to violence. Most recently, in a major outburst, he grabbed my mother's arm so hard that she is severely bruised. This scares me because I think of the future. How long will my mom be able to care for my brother? How am I supposed to take care of him in the future? There is no real plan for him and it is all going to fall on me. This is not fair to me. When I share my frustration with my wife, she withdraws from the conversation and reminds me that our kids come first. I feel so torn between the needs of both families. Nothing feels good or right.

Isolation Other feelings that siblings may experience tend to mirror those experienced by parents, such as loneliness and isolation (Calio & Higgins-D'Alessandro, 2021). These experiences are not uncommon for families with a disabled child due to social and societal barriers and the behavioral and care needs of the person with a disability. In younger siblings, feelings of embarrassment can result from their siblings actions being outside of societal norms, such as actions and outbursts, during public situations (D'Arcy et al., 2005) and can contribute to social isolation (Calio & Higgins-D'Alessandro, 2021).

A lack of social support is a significant concern across the lifespan of siblings. A lack of shared experiences with others can contribute to feelings of social isolation, as well as stress and other mental health experiences (Bellin & Kovacs, 2006; Simich et al., 2003). Siblings may choose not to discuss their feelings and experiences with their peers due to concerns regarding their response or their lack of understanding (Bellin & Kovacs, 2006; Hanvey et al., 2022; Simich et al., 2003) For example, a young child may not express how they became angry with their brother or sister to their peers for fear of being shamed for having feelings of anger toward their brother or sister with a disability. An older adult may not reach out to a peer to share a celebration in getting approved for a supportive service due to the peer not understanding the challenges that were present in receiving the service qualification. This lack of sharing and connection can cause siblings to internalize negative emotions and subsequently increase feelings of isolation and sadness (Hanvey et al., 2022) which can contribute to higher stress levels, depressive symptoms and feelings of being burdened (Saxena, 2015).

Supporting siblings through feelings of isolation is similar to those of parents. Connecting siblings to a community of peers with shared experiences is an excellent way to address isolation. Whether through informal connections such as family friends or through formal groups and curriculum-based programs, providing a community of support with like peers is one of the most effective ways to support siblings (Carter et al., 2016; Moyson & Roeyers, 2012; Naylor & Prescott, 2004).

I have two older sisters that are not involved, at all, with my twin. It's as if because she's "my twin" they take zero responsibility and expect me to handle everything for her since my parents have passed away. I feel so alone in this process. Over the years, I have tried to push them to have a relationship with my twin. I imagine she misses them and wonders where they are. I am setting up my twin's room at her residential home, trying to make it feel like home. I feel terrible but I don't even want to put pictures of my sisters in her room. Why bother? They don't bother at all.

It is sad but true. I hesitated to call home to share the great news with my parents about my career success. I recently received a bonus and a car allowance which affords me my very first, new car! I so wanted to share the news, but as I grabbed the phone to call them, I broke down in tears. I know that they can't be happy for me without comparing my life to the struggles my brother faces daily. I knew I'd have to minimize the happiness I feel so I've decided not to share this with them. I guess I'll have to explain the new car when they next see me. It won't feel good then, either. I feel so alone with my own successes and struggles.

Externalizing Behaviors

Externalizing behaviors may likely be due to the aforementioned emotional impacts and sense of responsibility (Brinkman et al., 2023: Giallo et al., 2012; Hayden et al., 2023; Knecht et al., 2014; Rochefort et al., 2023; Wolff et al., 2023). Given this, there is the potential for mental health conditions such as anxiety and depression to be present. The physical symptoms of anxiety in young children may take the form of somatic complaints (unexplained physical symptoms such as a headache, dizziness, or stomachache), shortness of breath, sweating or trembling, as well as general sleep disturbances such as difficulty staying asleep, nightmares, or restless sleep (Hooper, 2007; Stoneman, 2005). Symptoms of depression may include social withdrawal, lack of self-care, self-harm, and lack of desire to participate in family activities (Hooper, 2007; Stoneman, 2005).

The symptoms of anxiety and depression may manifest in behaviors such as avoidance/refusal to engage in school or other activities, clinginess, repetitive behaviors (counting, checking things), and emotional outbursts such as tantrums or emotional meltdowns due to fears and stress. Finally, young children especially may be prone to behavioral and emotional outbursts as they attempt to express their emotions and gain the attention of the parents even if the attention may not be in a positive form.

As a teen I would often start arguments with my mom. She always was so consumed with monitoring my sister's safety, coordinating her services, or attending her therapy appointments. As an adult, I can look back now and understand that my arguments were a plea for attention. I don't blame my mom for all the time that she spent on my sister, but I can see now that I also wanted attention but didn't quite know how to ask for it at the time. Now I can tell her that I'd like for it to only be the two of us for a lunch date.

Caregiving/Future Planning

The final challenge to be discussed is the caregiving role many adult siblings face as their parents age and are unable to fill this role. Most siblings plan to take on some sort of a care role with their brother or sister (Heller & Arnold, 2010; Heller & Kramer, 2009; Heller et al., 2008) and express concerns with taking on this role. Compounding this responsibility is the dual caregiving role that siblings may be faced with when caring for both their aging parents as well as their sibling (Lee et al., 2024).

Many factors will impact whether or not a sibling takes on a care role and to what extent they serve in this role. These factors include personal situations such as having poor relationships with their brother or sister, or with their parents (Burbidge & Minnes, 2014, Hodapp & Urbano, 2007; Saxena, 2015) or distance apart in living situations (Rimmerman, 2001). Notably even siblings who indicate a high level of satisfaction in their caregiver role, indicate the financial strain to be a challenge

(Saxena, 2015). Siblings report feelings of fear and uncertainty regarding their brother or sister's future care (Casale et al., 2021; Paul et al., 2022), especially in navigating the disability and social systems (Casale et al., 2021).

Siblings who indicate a greater satisfaction in taking on a caregiving role have had open communication within their family regarding future planning and caregiving roles (Marks et al., 2005). This open communication likely facilitates a more positive relationship between the siblings and their parents, thus supporting both the personal and practical needs of caregiving.

Other factors that influence a more positive caregiver role involve having a support network in place. When perceived support is low, siblings indicate higher stress levels, symptoms of depression and feelings of being burdened by the role (Saxena, 2015). Siblings that receive support from friends and family may continue in the caregiving responsibilities longer than those who do not perceive support (Saxena, 2015).

I finally mustered up the courage to talk to my parents about a transition plan for my sister. She is with them now, but they are seventy-five and it's only a matter of time before I am going to have to be the primary caregiver. What makes it even harder is that my sister isn't even connected to services or benefits, so I'll have to start from scratch when the time comes. This isn't new for me. As a kid, I was constantly expected to step in and help. Now, as an adult, I thought we could have a productive conversation about what's next. I shared how stressful this is for me, hoping for collaboration. Instead, my dad stopped speaking to me and my mom pretends nothing is wrong.

Everyone calls me "the black sheep" of the family. I am perfectly fine with that. The only way I knew I could survive and have my own life was to move as far as possible from my family. They recently invited me to meet with a special needs trust attorney with them. I wish they would understand that I have my own life and want nothing to do with planning for my brother. It is not my job; I am not his parent and don't care to fill this role in his life.

Recommendations for Supporting Siblings

Support for siblings, both young and old should center around the sibling feeling valued, seen and acknowledged. This can be accomplished by ensuring open communication (Marks et al., 2005), promoting healthy sibling relationships, fostering a community of support (Carter et al., 2016; Moyson & Roeyers, 2012), developing coping strategies (Orsmond & Seltzer, 2000), and ensuring the personal growth of the sibling. Siblings often garner attention from their role as a caregiver or because of their interactions with their brother or sister. For this reason, it is important to ensure there are opportunities for the sibling to also be validated for their personal interests and achievements as well so their sense of self worth is not attached to their role as a sibling.

Open communication can help siblings to express both positive and negative emotions. Many siblings may feel conflicted in feeling love and resentment toward their brother or sister. Creating a safe, accepting environment where all emotions can be expressed can help address issues of confusion that may arise with what seem to be conflicting emotions. Additionally, a parent that is educated on the experiences of siblings can have a positive impact on the sibling. This knowledge can facilitate awareness of and sensitivity to the needs of their non-disabled child, which in turn improves the overall health of the family system (Williams et al., 2022) Open communication can also provide age-appropriate information and an understanding around current and future care roles (Conway & Meyer, 2008; Hanvey et al., 2022). Many adult siblings indicate that involvement in future planning is beneficial (Saxena, 2015). Involvement in decision making can foster a sense of inclusion and purpose, especially given that most siblings will take on a care support role as their parents age.

Promoting healthy sibling relationships may take on different forms throughout the lifespan. Many issues that arise for young children, such as possessiveness around toys and sibling disagreements, will also be present for siblings with and without a disability. Ensuring the needs of all siblings are addressed should be the focus. Many siblings share frustration in having to be the accommodating child as parents may not hold their brother or sister to expectations that align with their ability (Drzymala et al., 2023). For example, when assisting with household duties, the disabled child does not have responsibilities even though they may have the ability to do tasks such as setting the table. Additionally, in the case of aggressive behavior in the home, siblings may have fear that would impede and limit their ability to engage in typical sibling interactions. For example, although it may seem feasible in the moment to have the typical sibling "give in" to the needs of the other (let them play with their toy so the other child doesn't become upset), such actions can foster feelings of resentment. Even though this may be appropriate on occasion, such as in any sibling relationship, adults should be sure to respect the needs of all children.

Adult sibling relationships may take on a variety of forms, from being a full-time live-in caregiver to minimal or no contact. In any case, respecting the wishes of the adult sibling is important. Typical siblings may choose to have close relationships just as they may choose to have a minimal relationship; either way the decision should be respected. Periodic check-ins or a general openness to conversations around family roles can be helpful to ensure a healthy relationship among all siblings in the family.

Many parents of young siblings and adult siblings opt to participate in therapeutic interventions. Counseling, therapy and other mental health support may be options for both youth and adult siblings. Interventions can be individual-focused and/or family-focused. Although not necessary, it may be helpful to ensure that the therapist understands the needs of families with both disabled and non-disabled children.

Community and Curriculum-Based Programs

The most recommended support mechanism for siblings, both young and old is a social network of peers that have shared experiences (Hanvey et al., 2022; Naylor &

Prescott, 2004; Simich et al., 2003). The social support provided through meaningful and supportive relationships has the potential to mitigate many of the concerns discussed such as social isolation, stress, mental health issues, and physical issues (Carter et al., 2016; Hanvey et al., 2022; Jones et al., 2020; Moyson & Roeyers, 2012; Simich et al., 2003; Wolff et al., 2023). Where secure peer relationships exist, children and adults may authentically express their thoughts, feelings, and behaviors (Hanvey et al., 2022; Naylor & Prescott, 2004).

There is currently no universal policy for supporting siblings (Saxena, 2015) with few programs in place to provide formal support and a pathway for social networks. Local and national disability organizations may offer support for siblings and include adult siblings in parent groups. The most prevalent sibling-focused intervention for youth is SibShops curriculum by the Sibling Support Project. This curriculum is developed for elementary aged children and brings young siblings together to provide recreational activities to facilitate information and peer support (Sibling Support Project, n.d.). Adults who participated in SibShops in their youth have indicated that their participation impacted their adult lives, taught them coping strategies, and had a positive impact on their feelings toward their sibling (Sibling Support Project, n.d.). Adults can become certified SibShop facilitators and host SibShops in their local area and/or via an online platform.

While SibShops are focused on supporting young siblings, the Sibling Leadership Network (SLN) focuses their efforts on adult siblings. The SLN provides a community of support, information, and resources for adult siblings (Sibling Leadership Network, n.d.). Many states host a state chapter of the SLN and collaborate for advocacy, policy change, and research to ensure the needs of siblings are included in discussions within the disability field, often collaborating with other local and state disability agencies (Sibling Leadership Network, n.d.). Additionally, the SLN hosts the virtual SibThrive program which is a curriculum-based cohort model group that is facilitated by a mental health professional sibling via online discussion that aims to create a community for discussion and understanding (Sibling Leadership Network, n.d.).

Effective support programs will include several key components: peer support and network building, discussion of feelings and emotions, coping strategies and problem-solving skills, identity and self-perception, and communication strategies (Calio & Higgins-D'Alessandro, 2021; Conway & Meyer, 2008; D'Arcy et al., 2005; Jones et al., 2020; Wolff et al., 2023). The most effective methodology for support programs is through a group format (Jones et al., 2020; Wolff et al., 2023) and may include some level of parental involvement and/or a parallel parental education component (Wolff et al., 2023). The above-mentioned SibShops and SibThrive programs include all of these components, with the exception of the parental involvement. However, although not part of the curriculum, parental education may be sought outside of the support programs.

Conclusion

Overall, adults report positive outcomes from being a sibling to a brother or sister with a disability and experience a long-lasting close relationship (Heller & Arnold, 2010). However, it is important to note that most research is conducted with female siblings and siblings that are engaged with their family; and more research is needed on siblings that are not engaged to garner a full perspective on the sibling experience. (Hanvey et al., 2022; Heller & Arnold, 2010). Based on what we know, families, friends and professionals providing a life span of support and communication around the sibling experience can help mitigate the challenges that arise. Most challenges that arise can be pre-empted by ensuring the siblings feel seen, heard and valued, even if this is facilitated through friends, family members, or other communities of support. Teaching siblings to develop and utilize coping strategies that focus on the specific problem can help develop perceptions of positivity and lower the perceived burden of providing care support (Saxena, 2015). Families, as well as those that support the families, can recognize and educate around the issues that may accompany being a sibling to someone with a disability and provide the support appropriate for their challenges (Hanvey et al., 2022).

Appendix

Scenarios and Possible Interventions

Scenario	Possible internalized feeling(s)	Possible externalized behavior(s)	Intervention
Mom, sibling and brother/sister with disability shopping at mall. Mom is distracted, stressed and preoccupied tending to sister's needs. Sibling left alone and is pressured to hurry and grab anything to wear without guidance	GLASS CHILD: Anxiety Insecurity Despair	Angry mannerisms, rushing, pretending to be okay despite frustrations, snappy voice tone "I'm fine!"	Develop state of curiosity of child's pain Understand there is no irrational outburst and seek to determine the deeper feelings of situation for child
Sibling asks to play game with dad. They are dismissed and told "no" because they are doing occupational therapy with sib	Feelings of rejection or not belonging	Withdraws to room or corner of room	Set timer for sib therapy hour that child can monitor, along with a promise for play when therapy is concluded

(continued)

(continued)

Scenario	Possible internalized feeling(s)	Possible externalized behavior(s)	Intervention
Mother overwhelmed and dealing with overwhelm of disabled child and challenged marriage	Feelings of loss of control or needing to control Anxiety of what needs to be done—unconscious anxious thought—"If I don't do it no one will."	Stepping in as adult lead role. Parentification	Gently redirect child to child-like role. Invite age-appropriate play, creativity, etc. Thank child's efforts but verbalize and clarify family role: "I am the mother. This is my job."
Sibling is hitting various milestones: Moving out of family home, graduating college, engagement, pregnancy	Guilt, concerns success will cause others pain. Wrestle with feelings of "not deserving"	Minimize personal triumphs, successes or achievements. May downplay or withhold information to prevent real or imagined pain, jealousy, or envy in others.	Invite celebratory conversations, be open and affirming around successes/ achievements. Encourage external therapeutic support to bolster a right to thrive in individual pursuits
Forgotten birthdays, missed pick-up/car pool, overlooked at tuck-in time, no breakfast prepared or school lunch ready to go	Neglect—Feeling unworthy of time and attention from caregivers due to their attending to the high demand/needs from brother or sister with disability	Unhealthy attention seeking behavior: Somaticize hurt. May engage in risky attention seeking behavior: theft, fighting, stealing, substance abuse, etc.	Notice cries for help and encourage expression of feelings. Calm, but firm parenting presence and parental accountability. Acknowledgment in repair for missed moments.
Sibling striving for straight A's, teacher's pet. Seeking validation for independent, activities such as, "I never have to worry about you"	Perfect child: Anxiety, perfectionism, neglect	Overachieving to compensate or relieve the family system of further overwhelm. Receives praise for success and low need.	Praise efforts but work to support, affirm and celebrate personal attributes more so than their productivity and accomplishments. Let them know it's okay to not be perfect.

References

Bellin, M. H., & Kovacs, P. J. (2006). Fostering resilience in siblings of youths with a chronic health condition: A review of the literature. *Health & Social Work, 31*(3), 209–216. https://doi.org/10.1093/hsw/31.3.209

Benson, P., & Karlof, K. L. (2008). Child, parent, and family predictors of latter adjustment in siblings of children with autism. *Research in Autism Spectrum Disorders, 2*, 583–600.

Bowen, M. (1966). The use of family theory in clinical practice. *Comprehensive Psychiatry, 7*, 345–374. https://doi.org/10.1016/s0010-440x(66)80065-2

Brinkman, A. H., Barry, T. D., & Lindsey, R. A. (2023). The relation of parental expressed emotion, parental affiliate stigma, and typically-developing sibling internalizing behavior in families with a child with ASD. *Journal of Autism and Developmental Disorders, 53*, 4591–4603. https://doi.org/10.1007/s10803-022-05760-3

Burbidge, J., & Minnes, P. (2014). Relationship quality in adult siblings with and without developmental disabilities. *Family Relations, 63*(1), 148–162. https://doi.org/10.1111/fare.12047

Calio, C., & Higgins-D'Alessandro, A. (2021). "It's really unexplainable, but everyone here got it:" Analysis of an ASD sibling support group for emerging adults. *Research in Autism Spectrum Disorders, 88*, 101857. https://doi.org/10.1016/j.rasd.2021.101857

Carr, J. (2005). Families of 30-35-year olds with down's syndrome. *Journal of Applied Research in Intellectual Disabilities, 18*, 75–84. https://doi.org/10.1111/j.1468-3148.2004.00226.x

Carter, S., Cook, J., Sutton-Boulton, G., Ward, V., & Clarke, S. (2016). Social pedagogy as a model to provide support for siblings of children with intellectual disabilities: A report of the views of the children and young people using a sibling support group. *Journal of Intellectual Disabilities, 20*(1), 65–81. https://doi.org/10.1177/1744629515586516

Casale, E. G., Burke, M. M., Urbano, R. C., Arnold, C. K., & Hodapp, R. M. (2021). Getting from here to there: Future planning as reported by adult siblings of individuals with disabilities. *Journal of Intellectual Disability Research, 65*(3), 246–261. https://doi.org/10.1111/jir.12806

Conway, S., & Meyer, D. (2008). Developing support for siblings of young people with disabilities. *Support for Learning, 23*(3), 113–117. https://doi.org/10.1111/j.1467-9604.2008.00381.x

D'Arcy, F., Flynn, J., McCarthy, Y., O'Connor, C., & Tierney, E. (2005). Sibshops: An evaluation of an interagency model. *Journal of Intellectual Disabilities, 9*(1), 43–57. https://doi.org/10.1177/1744629505049729

Drzymala, H., Grey, B., & Fowler, N. (2023). Exploring the triadic parent-child-sibling relationship: How do mothers' view of their child impact sibling relationships? *Human Systems: Therapy, Culture and Attachments, 3*(2), 92–111. https://doi.org/10.1177/26344041221145619

Giallo, R., Gavidia-payne, S., Minett, B., & Kapoor, A. (2012). Sibling voices: The self-reported mental health of siblings of children with a disability. *Clinical Psychologist, 16*(1), 36–43. https://doi.org/10.1111/j.1742-9552.2011.00035.x

Hanvey, I., Malovic, A., & Ntontis, E. (2022). Glass children: The lived experiences of siblings of people with a disability or chronic illness. *Journal of Community & Applied Social Psychology, 32*. https://doi.org/10.1002/casp.2602

Hayden, N. K., Hastings, R. P., & Bailey, T. (2023). Behavioural adjustment of children with intellectual disability and their sibling is associated with their sibling relationship quality. *Journal of Intellectual Disability Research, 67*(4), 310–322. https://doi.org/10.1111/jir.13006

Heller, T., & Arnold, K. (2010). Siblings of adults with developmental disabilities: Psychosocial outcomes, relationships, and future planning. *Journal of Policy and Practice in Intellectual Disabilities., 7*, 16–25. https://doi.org/10.1111/j.1741-1130.2010.00243.x

Heller, T., & Kramer, J. (2009). Involvement of adult siblings of people with developmental disabilities in future planning. *Intellectual and Developmental Disabilities, 47*, 208–219. https://doi.org/10.1352/1934-9556-47.3.208

Heller, T., Kaiser, A., Meyer, D., Fish, T., Kramer, J., & Dufresne, D. (2008). The sibling leadership network: Recommendations for research, advocacy, and supports relating to siblings of people with developmental disabilities. Retrieved from https://siblingleadership.org/wp-content/uploads/2013/02/SLN-White-Paper-Final-2.pdf

Hodapp, R. M., & Urbano, R. C. (2007). Adult siblings of individuals with Down syndrome versus with autism: Findings from a large-scale US survey. *Journal of Intellectual Disability Research, 51*, 1018–1029. https://doi.org/10.1111/j.1365-2788.2007.00994.x

Hooper, L. M. (2007). The application of attachment theory and family systems theory to the phenomenon of parentification. *The Family Journal, 15*(3), 217–223. https://doi.org/10.1177/1066480707301290

Jajodia, P., & Roy, P. (2023). Sibling issues in disability: A thematic analysis of sibling, parent & expert perspectives. *International Journal of Disability, Development and Education, 70*(7), 1392–1409. https://doi.org/10.1080/1034912X.2022.2060948

Jones, E., Fiani, T., Stewart, J., Neil, N., McHugh, S., & Fienup, D. (2020). Randomized controlled trial of a sibling support group: Mental health outcomes for siblings of children with autism. *Autism, 24*(6), 1468–1481. https://doi.org/10.1177/13623613209089

Kaminsky, L., & Dewey, D. (2002). Psychosocial adjustment in siblings of children with autism. *Journal of Child Psychology & Psychiatry & Allied Disciplines, 43*(2), 225–233.

Knecht, C., Hellmers, C., & Metzing, S. (2014). The perspective of siblings of children with chronic illness A literature review. *Journal of Pediatric Nursing, 30*(1), 102–116. https://doi.org/10.1016/j.pedn.2014.10.010

Kovacs, T., Possick, C., & Buchbinder, E. (2019). Experiencing the relationship with a sibling coping with mental health problems: Dilemmas of connection, communication, and role. *Health and Social Care in the Community, 27*, 1185–1192. https://doi.org/10.1111/hsc.12761

Lee, C. E., Hagiwara, M., Burke, M. M., & Arnold, C. K. (2024). Family support and disability policies: Perspectives of siblings of people with intellectual and developmental disabilities. *Journal of Disability Policy Studies*. https://doi.org/10.1177/10442073241289088

Liu, J., Chen, X., & Lewis, G. (2011). Childhood internalizing behaviour: Analysis and implications. *Journal of Psychiatric and Mental Health Nursing, 18*(10), 884–894. https://doi.org/10.1111/j.1365-2850.2011.01743.x

Lobato, D., Kao, B., & Plante, W. (2011). Psychological and school functioning of latino siblings of children with intellectual disability. *Journal of Child Psychology and Psychiatry, 52*(6), 696–703. https://doi.org/10.1111/j.1469-7610.2010.02357.x

Marks, S. U., Matson, A., & Barraza, L. (2005). The impact of siblings with disabilities on their brothers and sisters pursuing a career in special education. *Research & Practice for Persons with Severe Disabilities, 30*(4), 205–218. https://doi.org/10.2511/rpsd.30.4.205

Marquis, S. M., McGrail, K., & Hayes, M. V. (2019). A population-level study of the mental health of siblings of children who have a developmental disability. *SSM - Population Health, 28*(8). https://doi.org/10.1016/j.ssmph.2019.100441

McGraw, L. A., & Walker, A. J. (2007). Meanings of sisterhood and developmental disability: Narratives from white nondisabled sisters. *Journal of Family Issues, 28*(4), 474–500. https://doi.org/10.1177/0192513x06297312

Moyson, T., & Roeyers, H. (2012). "The overall quality of my life as a sibling is all right, but of course, it could always be better". Quality of life of siblings of children with intellectual disability: The siblings' perspectives. *Journal of Intellectual Disability Research, 56*(1), 87–101. https://doi.org/10.1111/j.1365-2788.2011.01393.x

Naylor, A., & Prescott, P. (2004). Invisible children? The need for support groups for siblings of disabled children. *British Journal of Special Education, 31*, 199–206. https://doi.org/10.1111/j.0952-3383.2004.00355.x

Neece, C. L., Blacher, J., & Baker, B. L. (2010). Impact on siblings of children with intellectual disability: The role of child behavior problems. *American Journal on Intellectual and Developmental Disabilities, 115*(4), 291–306. https://doi.org/10.1352/1944-7558-115.4.291

Orm, S., Haukeland, Y., Vatne, T., Silverman, W. K., & Fjermestad, K. (2022). Prosocial behavior is a relative strength in siblings of children with physical disabilities or autism spectrum disorder. *Journal of Developmental & Physical Disabilities, 34*(4), 591–608. https://doi.org/10.1007/s10882-021-09816-7

Orsmond, G., & Seltzer, M. (2000). Brothers and sisters with mental retardation: Gendered nature of the sibling relationship. *American Journal of Mental Retardation, 105*(6), 486–508. https://doi.org/10.1352/0895-8017(2006)111[155:MOCSOD]2.0.CO;2

Paul, A. M., Hussey, M. M., Woodman, A. C., Smith, A. L., & Shriver, T. P. (2022). Experiences of siblings of people with intellectual disabilities: Multiregional perspectives. *Family Relations, 71*(2), 671–685. https://doi.org/10.1111/fare.12608

Rimmerman, A. (2001). Involvement with and role perception toward an adult sibling with and without mental retardation. *Journal of Rehabilitation, 67*(2), 10–15.

Rixon, L., Hastings, R. P., & Kovshoff, H. (2025). It feels very weird and normal at the same time': Sibling perceptions of their relationships with an autistic brother of sister with complex care needs. *Journal of Applied Research in Intellectual Disabilities, 38*(1). https://doi.org/10.1111/jar.70009

Rochefort, C., Paradis, A., Rivard, M., & Dewar, M. (2023). Siblings of individuals with intellectual disabilities or autism: A scoping review using trauma theory. *Journal of Child and Family Studies, 32*(11), 3482–3500. https://doi.org/10.1007/s10826-023-02589-x

Rodger, S., & Tooth, L. (2004). Adult siblings' perceptions of family life and loss: A pilot case study. *Journal of Developmental and Physical Disabilities, 16*(1), 53–71. https://doi.org/10.1023/B:JODD.0000010039.14986.41

Rossiter, L., & Sharpe, D. (2001). The siblings of individuals with mental retardation: A quantitative integration of the literature. *Journal of Child and Family Studies, 10*(1), 65–84. https://doi.org/10.1023/a:1016629500708

Saxena, M. (2015). Variables that can enhance and complicate sibling caregiving of individuals with intellectual and developmental disabilities. *Journal of Policy and Practice in Intellectual Disabilities, 12*(3), 210–219. https://doi.org/10.1111/jppi.12127

Saxena, M., & Adamsons, K. (2013). Siblings of individuals with disabilities: Reframing the literature through a bioecological lens. *Journal of Family Theory & Review, 5*(4), 300–316. https://doi.org/10.1111/jftr.12021

Seltzer, M. M., Krauss, M. W., Hong, J., & Orsmond, G. I. (2001). Continuity or discontinuity of family involvement following residential transitions of adults who have mental retardation. *Mental Retardation, 39*(3), 181–194. https://doi.org/10.1352/0047-6765(2001)039<0181:CODOFI>2.0.CO;2

Sibling Leadership Network. (n.d.). https://www.siblingleadership.org

Sibling Support Project. (n.d.). https://www.siblingsupport.org

Simich, L., Beiser, M., & Mawani, F. N. (2003). Social support and the significance of shared experience in refugee migration and resettlement. *Western Journal of Nursing Research, 25*(7), 872–891. https://doi.org/10.1177/0193945903256705

Stoneman, Z. (2005). Siblings of children with disabilities: Research themes. *Mental Retardation, 43*(5), 339–350. https://doi.org/10.1352/0047-6765(2005)43[339:SOCWDR]2.0.CO;2

Taylor, T. M., Roper, S. O., Woodruff, M., Grow, H. P., & Freeborn, D. (2023). Family cohesion and positive sibling relationships in families raising a child with or without a disability. *Exceptionality, 31*(2), 118–134. https://doi.org/10.1080/09362835.2022.2100391

TEDx Talks. (2010, December 27). EDxSanAntonio—Alicia Arenas—Recognising Glass Children [Video] Youtube. https://www.youtube.com/watch?v=MSwqo-g2Tbk

Tomeny, T. S., Barry, T. D., & Fair, E. C. (2017). Parentification of adult siblings of individuals with autism spectrum disorder: Distress, sibling relationship attitudes, and role of social support. *Journal of Intellectual & Developmental Disability, 42*(4), 320–331. https://doi.org/10.3109/13668250.2016.1248376

Williams, C. A., Bailey, T., & Hastings, R. P. (2022). Modelling triadic relationships in families of children with intellectual disability. *Journal of Applied Research in Intellectual Disabilities, 35*(3), 843–855. https://doi.org/10.1111/jar.12988

Wolff, B., Magiati, I., Roberts, R., Skoss, R., & Glasson, E. J. (2023). Psychosocial interventions and support groups for siblings of individuals with neurodevelopmental conditions: A mixed methods systematic review of sibling self-reported mental health and wellbeing outcomes. *Clinical Child and Family Psychology Review, 26*(1), 143–189. https://doi.org/10.1007/s10567-022-00413-4

Chapter 7
Role of the Family in Promoting Success for Children with Developmental Disabilities and Health Conditions

Kimberly R. Tomeny and Robin A. McWilliam

Abstract This chapter examines the essential role of families in fostering development, inclusion, and resilience in children with developmental disabilities and health conditions. Drawing from Family Systems and Ecological Systems theories, it emphasizes family-centered practice and advocates for collaborative, strengths-based partnerships between families and professionals. The chapter highlights evidence-based interventions, including caregiver-implemented strategies and coaching, that empower families to support child learning in daily routines. Components such as collaboration, feedback, problem solving, and routine-based learning are illustrated through early intervention models. The authors underscore improved child engagement, communication, functional skills, and caregiver competence as key outcomes of family capacity-building. The chapter also discusses advocacy, cultural responsiveness, and resource access, stressing the importance of practitioners honoring family priorities. By centering families in intervention planning, the chapter argues practitioners can strengthen child and family outcomes, and calls for continuous evaluation and adoption of family-centered, evidence-based practices.

Keywords Family · Children with developmental disabilities · Family-centered practice · Caregiver coaching strategies · Caregiver-implemented interventions · Caregiving practices

Families play a crucial role in supporting the development of young children (Bronfenbrenner, 1974; Dunst & Trivette, 2014). Leading early childhood organizations, such as the Division for Early Childhood (DEC, 2014) of the Council for Exceptional Children (CEC) and the National Association for the Education of Young Children

K. R. Tomeny (✉)
Department of Human Development and Family Studies, University of Alabama, Tuscaloosa, AL, USA
e-mail: krtomeny@ua.edu

R. A. McWilliam
Department of Special Education, University of Alabama, Tuscaloosa, AL, USA

L. Nabors and T. Stanton-Chapman (eds.), *Developmental Disabilities and Chronic Illness in Young Children*, Springer Series on Child and Family Studies,
https://doi.org/10.1007/978-3-032-08523-8_7

(NAEYC, 2020), emphasize the importance of partnering with families in these organizations' evidence-based guidelines for working with young children, including those with disabilities. To enhance families' confidence and competence, experts recommend that practitioners across disciplines include families of young children with disabilities and health conditions in the various aspects of their work, such as decision-making, outcome development, and intervention delivery (DEC, 2014; McWilliam, 2010b). Through implementation of evidence-based practices aimed at building family capacity, practitioners can support families of young children as "a primary source of influence on child behavior, learning, and development" (Dunst & Espe-Sherwindt, 2016, p. 37).

Family-Centered Practice

Family-centered practice is an approach that focuses on empowering families by emphasizing strengths, building capacity, and fostering collaboration to promote positive child and family outcomes (Dunst, 2002; Dunst & Trivette, 2014). As Bailey et al. (2012) note, when taking a family-centered approach, it is necessary for practitioners to view the child within the context of the family, because services cannot be provided appropriately without such consideration. Family systems theory (Bowen, 1966) and ecological systems theory (Bronfenbrenner, 1974) support this line of thinking, such that children are part of a larger family unit whereby caregivers can influence child functioning (and vice versa). Consider your own upbringing, for example, and the many ways in which your family might have influenced your growth, development, and learning (as well as how you might have influenced the overall functioning of your family unit). Viewing the child outside of the family unit provides only a small snapshot of the larger picture and neglects the important role families play in shaping their children's lives. Thus, taking a family-centered approach to working with young children offers a holistic representation of what a child's life truly looks like and conveys how significant families are in supporting their children (now and throughout their lives).

Professional organizations across different fields (e.g., special education, occupational therapy, physical therapy, speech-language pathology, medicine) endorse family-centered practice in their personnel competencies and recommended practices, emphasizing the value and importance of this approach, regardless of disciplinary background (Bailey et al., 2012; Bruder et al., 2019; DEC, 2014). In addition, research findings support the use of family-centered practice across disciplines for practitioners working with children with developmental disabilities and health conditions. For example, several meta-analyses and systematic literature reviews show an association between practitioners' implementation of family-centered practices and positive outcomes for children and families. Such outcomes include improvements in child health, child psychological outcomes, caregiver-child interactions, caregiver well-being, use of evidence-based parenting practices, family relationships, and family functioning (Dunst et al., 2007; Dunst & Trivette, 2009; Kuhlthau et al., 2011;

McBroom & Enriquez, 2009). Thus, the emphasis on family-centeredness in practitioners' everyday practice is widely recommended and accepted as an evidence-based approach to working with young children with disabilities and health conditions, as well as their families.

Specific Family-Centered Intervention Practices

Working with families of young children can be challenging at times, because each family is different and has unique priorities and concerns specific to their individual circumstances. Knowledge and understanding of specific family-centered intervention practices is the first step in helping practitioners develop their ability to make family-centeredness a core component of their practice. As mentioned previously, DEC (2014) provides research-based guidance for effective ways to engage with families and support young children with disabilities, developmental delays, and health conditions. Table 7.1 outlines family-centered practices from DEC's (2014) Recommended Practices, with specific examples of what they look like and what they do not look like.

Evidence-Based Interventions

In addition to specific family-centered practices that practitioners can embed into their work with families, different evidence-based models and approaches to intervention exist, designed to support families of young children with disabilities and health conditions. These models and approaches incorporate the key principles of family-centered practice highlighted previously, emphasizing the importance of building families' capacity, competence, and confidence. The following sections provide an overview of family-centered models and approaches most commonly used in early childhood.

Family-Centered Models and Approaches in Early Intervention

Even though this book primarily addresses working with children ages 3 and above, some of the most influential work on family-centeredness comes from the early intervention literature, so it is essential to highlight research focused on infants and toddlers when discussing family-centered practice. Beyond general recommendations, federal legislation under Part C of the Individuals with Disabilities Education Act (IDEA, 2004) requires early intervention providers in the United States to use family-centered practices when delivering services to infants and toddlers

Table 7.1 Using family-centered intervention practices with families of young children

DEC recommended practice	What it looks like	What it doesn't look like
F1. Practitioners build trusting and respectful partnerships with the family through interactions that are sensitive and responsive to cultural, linguistic, and socio-economic diversity.	Building rapport with families	Working only with the child
	Engaging in respectful interactions with families	Talking down to families
	Responding to families' diverse backgrounds	Assuming families have the same background as the practitioner
F2. Practitioners provide the family with up-to-date, comprehensive and unbiased information in a way that the family can understand and use to make informed choices and decisions.	Sharing current and accurate information with families	Providing families with dated and inaccurate information
	Providing families with information in a way that is easy to understand	Providing families with information using professional or technical jargon
F3. Practitioners are responsive to the family's concerns, priorities, and changing life circumstances.	Responding to and addressing families' priorities and concerns	Addressing practitioner's concerns
	Recognizing families' unique situations	Treating all families alike
F4. Practitioners and the family work together to create outcomes or goals, develop individualized plans, and implement practices that address the family's priorities and concerns and the child's strengths and needs.	Collaborating with families to determine outcomes, plans, and intervention strategies	Determining outcomes, plans, and intervention strategies for the family and child
	Addressing family functioning, in addition to child functioning	Addressing only child skills
F5. Practitioners support family functioning, promote family confidence and competence, and strengthen family-child relationships by acting in ways that recognize and build on family strengths and capacities.	Using a strengths-based approach to build family competence and confidence	Addressing perceived family weaknesses
	Encouraging positive interactions among children and family members	Working on child skills without addressing interactions in the family
F6. Practitioners engage the family in opportunities that support and strengthen parenting knowledge and skills and parenting competence and confidence in ways that are flexible, individualized, and tailored to the family's preferences.	Building family members' knowledge and skills	Working only with the child
	Addressing each family's individual priorities flexibly	Working with all families in the same way
F7. Practitioners work with the family to identify, access, and use formal and informal resources and supports to achieve family-identified outcomes or goals.	Connecting families to resources	Working only as a teacher, interventionist, or therapist, assuming someone else will connect families to resources

(continued)

Table 7.1 (continued)

DEC recommended practice	What it looks like	What it doesn't look like
F8. Practitioners provide the family of a young child who has or is at risk for developmental delay/disability, and who is a dual-language learner, with information about the benefits of learning in multiple languages for the child's growth and development.	Sharing information about benefits of dual-language learning	Addressing only single-language learning
F9. Practitioners help families know and understand their rights.	Clearly communicating families' rights	Not communicating families' rights
	Answering questions about families' rights	Failing to get answers to families' questions about their rights
F10. Practitioners inform families about leadership and advocacy skill-building opportunities and encourage those who are interested to participate.	Encouraging family involvement in leadership and advocacy	Addressing families' roles as caregivers only, not as potential leaders or advocates

Adapted from DEC's Recommended Practices, 2014

(i.e., birth to 3 years) with developmental delays and disabilities. Different evidence-based models and approaches to family-centered early intervention exist, including the Routines-Based Model of Early Intervention Birth to Five (RBM; McWilliam, 2010a), Family Guided Routines-Based Intervention (FGRBI; Woods, 2024), and the coaching approach (Rush & Shelden, 2019). While these models and approaches consist of varying components and practices, they also share similarities in ways in which they include, support, empower, and collaborate with families, incorporating evidence-based, family-centered practices into their service delivery.

Given the federal requirements that guide the use of family-centered practices in early intervention for children under 3 years of age, early intervention lends itself to serving as an example of how to include families meaningfully into one's practice for the broader community of practitioners who interact with young children with developmental disabilities and health conditions. We argue that a child's family is just as important when the child turns 3 as they were before the child's third birthday, whether legislative requirements for family-centered practice exist or not. Thus, practitioners should include families in services throughout a child's life, not solely in infancy and toddlerhood (McWilliam, 2010b). Later in this chapter, we describe examples from one of the family-centered models in early intervention, the RBM, as an illustration of the practical application of family-centered practice.

Caregiver-Implemented Intervention

Caregiver-implemented intervention (also described as *caregiver-mediated intervention, parent-implemented intervention,* or *parent-mediated intervention*) is a foundational component of family-centered practice, providing guidance for the inclusion of children's families in service delivery (Movahedazarhouligh, 2021). Caregiver-implemented intervention is an evidence-based approach that supports caregivers to facilitate their child's learning and development in everyday routines, often guided through practitioners' use of caregiver coaching strategies (Pellecchia et al., 2024; Romano et al., 2022; Tomeny et al., 2020; Wong et al., 2015). In recent years, practitioners have increasingly used caregiver-implemented intervention as an approach to working with families of young children with confirmed or suspected delays or disabilities (Movahedazarhouligh, 2021; Pellecchia et al., 2024).

Experts and practitioners recognize the value of caregivers' natural involvement in children's everyday activities and routines, where learning and development most often occur in early childhood (Barton & Fettig, 2013; Romano et al., 2022). For example, consider what mealtimes might look like for a young child, thinking about the many potential learning opportunities and the interactions that might occur between the child and their typical caregiver. By taking a caregiver-implemented intervention approach, practitioners can promote these optimal learning opportunities and interactions by building on what is already occurring and supporting the caregiver within this context (Swanson et al., 2011).

In caregiver-implemented intervention, we can think of the caregiver as the person in the driver's seat, rather than the practitioner. The caregiver should be the primary person interacting with the child while the practitioner coaches the caregiver to guide these caregiver-child interactions. Caregiver-implemented intervention focuses on supporting caregivers to use specific strategies with their children during the many hours they spend together throughout the week (McWilliam & Scott, 2001; Romano et al., 2022). Because children spend a significant amount of time engaging in their everyday routines with their natural caregivers, families can optimize that time and take advantage of the learning opportunities that are naturally occurring in their child's life. This looks different from having families set aside designated time for learning, which is often unnatural for learning in early childhood and not part of a child and family's everyday routine. Thus, in caregiver-implemented intervention, a practitioner's session time with the child and family should be spent preparing the caregivers for the time when the practitioner is *not* present. The components of caregiver-implemented intervention might be a shift in thinking for some practitioners who are accustomed to using session time to work directly with the child and take the lead in interactions with children and families; however, it is an important shift to make when using family-centered practices and facilitating caregiver-implemented intervention.

Research on caregiver-implemented intervention demonstrates the effectiveness of its use with families of children with various disabilities and developmental delays (Akemoglu & Meadan, 2018; Cheng et al., 2023; Heidlage et al., 2020;

Roberts & Kaiser, 2011). Results from studies examining the use of caregiver-implemented intervention show positive outcomes for caregivers, including caregivers' use of intervention strategies (Akemoglu & Meadan, 2018; Cheng et al., 2022; Roberts & Kaiser, 2011; Windsor et al., 2019). Studies also show improvements in child outcomes across domains, including cognition, language and communication, social functioning, behavior, daily living skills, and academic skills (Akemoglu & Meadan, 2018; Cheng et al., 2023; Green et al., 2010; Heidlage et al., 2020; Kasari et al., 2014; Rogers et al., 2012; Stadnick et al., 2015). Owing to the evidence and the family-centered nature of this approach, caregiver-implemented intervention is recommended when working with young children and their families.

Caregiver Coaching Strategies As mentioned previously, practitioners commonly use caregiver coaching strategies when taking a caregiver-implemented approach to intervention. Before diving further into caregiver coaching strategies, it is important to note that different terms exist in the literature to describe the process of supporting caregivers via caregiver-implemented intervention. For example, some refer to *collaborative consultation* (McWilliam, 2010b; Woods et al., 2011). Proponents of the term *coaching*, however, often use it to describe both an interaction approach with children's caregivers and to describe the process of training professionals (Kemp & Turnbull, 2014). In this chapter, we use the term *caregiver coaching* to refer to the practitioner's interactions with a child's primary caregivers as a means of facilitating caregiver-implemented intervention.

As Rogers et al. (2021) note, coaching caregivers to use intervention strategies with their children in their natural environments promotes increased child learning opportunities and fosters interactions with their caregivers. Similar to various models and approaches in early intervention, specific caregiver-implemented intervention models exist, each consisting of unique components. Despite these unique components, researchers have found common elements of caregiver coaching from the existing literature (Pellecchia et al., 2024; Tomeny et al., 2020). Pellecchia et al. (2024) conducted a scoping review of five specific caregiver coaching strategies, derived from existing research (Friedman et al., 2012, Kemp & Turnbull, 2014; Trivette et al., 2009), to determine the presence of these strategies in the manuals of different caregiver-implemented intervention models for young children with autism (birth to 8 years). Many of the existing caregiver-implemented intervention models focus on a specific disability (e.g., autism, deafness), with much of the caregiver-implemented intervention research to date conducted with autistic children and their families. The five caregiver coaching strategies Pellecchia et al. (2024) highlight include (a) collaboration, (b) daily routines, (c) demonstration, (d) feedback, and (e) reflection and problem solving. Table 7.2 provides a description of each caregiver coaching strategy with examples of what it looks like and what it does not look like.

Table 7.2 Caregiver coaching strategies

Caregiver coaching strategy	Description	What it looks like	What it doesn't look like
Collaboration	"Actively including the [caregiver] in developing intervention goals for their child and family and in deciding how to work on those goals."	Joint goal setting	Practitioner goal setting
		Caregivers making decisions during sessions	Practitioners making decisions during sessions
		Use of language that suggests practitioner/ caregiver team	Use of non-collaborative language
Daily routines	"Teaching [caregivers] to deliver the intervention directly in the environment or setting where it will ultimately be used."	Working on communication skills during mealtime	Working on communication skills during a "communication session"
		Supporting motor skills during outings to the playground the family frequently visits	Supporting motor skills by repeatedly walking back and forth on a balance beam
Demonstration	"Teaching [caregivers] to use an intervention strategy by modeling the use of an intervention strategy for a [caregiver] and explaining how to use the specific procedure."	Explicitly teaching a strategy to the caregiver	Implementing a strategy with the child without any explanation to the caregiver
		Explaining the purpose of a strategy to the caregiver	
		Explaining useful strategies to promote caregiver-child interaction	
Feedback	"Giving the [caregiver] an opportunity to practice the demonstrated technique and offering feedback about the [caregiver's] observed use of the technique."	Commenting on strategies that are working well	Not identifying what's working well
		Allowing sufficient time for the caregiver to practice a strategy	Not allowing opportunity for the caregiver to practice a strategy
		Providing constructive feedback	Being critical

(continued)

Table 7.2 (continued)

Caregiver coaching strategy	Description	What it looks like	What it doesn't look like
Reflection and problem solving	"Ask[ing] the [caregiver] to reflect on the use of an intervention strategy (after demonstration and feedback) and any potential barriers to using the strategy within daily routines. The provider and [caregiver] then collaborate on potential strategies to overcome any identified barriers."	Listening to caregiver concerns	Now allowing opportunity for caregiver to express concerns
		Collaboratively evaluating child's progress	Evaluating child's progress independently
		Helping the caregiver work through barriers to implementing a strategy	Only telling the caregiver what to do

Adapted from Pellecchia et al., 2024

The Need for Further Research and Evidence-Based Practice

Despite best-practice recommendations for working with families of young children with disabilities and health conditions across disciplines, the need for further research and evidence-based practice remains. Researchers note that evidence-based interventions do not always reach children and families in the community as intended, and they have called for changes to future research with the goal of addressing this issue (Rieth et al., 2018; Romano & Schnurr, 2022). Practitioners' application of research recommendations into their daily practice in the real world is commonly referred to as translation of research to practice. When challenges arise, a research-to-practice gap is revealed. Romano and Schnurr (2022) highlight the research-to-practice gap that exists around the use of family-centered practice and caregiver-implemented intervention approaches in early childhood. In the following sections, we discuss the implementation gap that commonly occurs in community-based settings and emphasize the importance of using evidence-based practice when working with families.

Research-to-Practice Gap

For many years, when attempting to translate research into practice, practitioners have faced challenges in being family centered. Results from numerous studies reveal a gap between recommendations informed by research and practitioners' actual practices (via report or observation) when working with families of young children (Campbell & Sawyer, 2007, 2009; Douglas et al., 2020; Peterson et al., 2007; Sawyer & Campbell, 2017). Research shows that practitioners tend to use practices that are less family-centered, with a focus on working directly with the child rather than spending session time coaching the caregiver via caregiver-implemented intervention (Douglas et al., 2020; Griffith et al., 2023; Peterson et al., 2007; Sawyer & Campbell, 2017). For example, in a study that examined video recordings of community-based intervention sessions, practitioners spent more than half of the time working directly with the child without explaining to the caregiver what they were doing (Sawyer & Campbell, 2017). In another study, practitioners shared their perceptions and experiences surrounding caregiver coaching, and results demonstrated limited use of certain caregiver coaching strategies, despite their reports of perceived importance of such strategies (Douglas et al., 2020). Practitioners who participated in this study also identified numerous challenges and barriers to coaching caregivers, including difficulties with caregiver engagement, language barriers, time constraints, and scheduling (Douglas et al., 2020). Similarly, findings from other studies have revealed challenges for practitioners and administrators when it comes to involving families in their practice (Movahedazarhouligh & Banerjee, 2020; Stein et al., 2025), adding potential explanation for the research-to-practice gap.

Despite the gap that exists between recommended and actual practice, practitioners and families generally agree on the importance of family-centered practices, acknowledging that such practices are recommended when working with young children (Crais et al., 2006; Kim et al., 2025; McWilliam, 2000). In addition, practitioners report that they value caregiver coaching and have positive attitudes surrounding evidence-based practice (Douglas et al., 2020; Griffith et al., 2023). Over the past few decades, however, numerous studies have shown a discrepancy between what practitioners report as typical practices and ideal practices across various components of the intervention process, including assessment, plan development, and service delivery (Bailey et al., 1992; Crais et al., 2006; Douglas et al., 2020; García-Ventura et al., 2021; McWilliam, 2000). Findings from such studies show that even when practitioners demonstrate awareness of ideal or recommended practices in their field, they do not always use such practices in their own work with families.

Results from a more recent study showed closer alignment between practitioners' ratings of typical and ideal practices related to family-centeredness, with less-significant differences between what practitioners commonly implement and what they consider as ideal (Tomeny et al., 2021). Whereas practitioners rated typical and ideal practices fairly highly overall, findings highlighted a large discrepancy between their typical and ideal ratings specific to working with the child or caregiver. For this item, practitioners generally reported that they recognized working with the caregiver as ideal practice, yet they were less likely to do so in their typical practice, demonstrating a gap specific to practices that facilitate caregiver-implemented intervention (Tomeny et al., 2021). Findings from the studies described above reveal that a gap not only exists between recommended and actual practice, but that practitioners are aware of this discrepancy by acknowledging the ways in which their own practices differ from what they consider to be ideal practice.

Even though gaps remain when it comes to implementation of evidence-based practice in the community, it is essential for practitioners to use evidence-based practice when working with young children and their families. Later in this chapter, we address the limitations of current research and make recommendations for changes to support increased use of evidence-based practice in community settings.

Promoting Successful Inclusion and Resilience in Children

A theme running through evidence-based practice in working with families is the role of families on children's inclusion and on their resilience. Arguably, families play the most important role in inclusion and resilience for young children. Here, we address three conditions or activities families can have, affecting this role. We provide examples from the internationally implemented Routines-Based Model (RBM) (McWilliam, 2000, 2010a, 2016) to demonstrate how these conditions or activities might look when embedded in service delivery.

First, we address the condition of receiving services such as early intervention, early childhood special education, and related services (e.g., therapy, medical services). When these services are designed to build the caregiver's capacity, caregivers such as parents and classroom teachers are emboldened to support the child in meaningful participation in daily routines (Dunst & Trivette, 2014). These routines might be times of day at home (e.g., breakfast time, hanging-out time, bathtime) or classroom routines (e.g., morning meeting time, free play time, snack time, outside time). If practitioners work with caregivers using collaborative consultation or caregiver coaching versus expert consultation, caregivers assume ownership over the interventions or strategies and are more likely to implement them between practitioners' visits (Shelden & Rush, 2022). For example, in the RBM, practitioners are trained to understand that the purpose of early intervention is to build caregivers' capacity, and they fulfill this role by implementing manualized Routines-Based Home Visits (McWilliam, 2012) and Collaborative Consultation to Children's Classrooms (Boavida et al., 2022).

A second activity is advocacy. Practitioners can educate families on their rights under IDEA (2004) and on resources (e.g., federally funded parent training and advocacy centers, parent groups, disability-specific organizations). Families can advocate for opportunities and services. When families advocate for an ineffective model of service delivery or a nonevidence-based treatment, practitioners need to share information with families objectively and explain gently why the system will not provide that service, all without passing judgment on families. Families almost always have some level of advocacy for their child through the IFSP or IEP process, but families have a history of advocating for children with disabilities beyond only their own child (Cunconan-Lahr & Brotherson, 1996). The RBM has some aphorisms practitioners are expected to know and abide by. Some of those related to advocacy are (a) *We have an ethical obligation to provide families with information* (e.g., about what practices are based in evidence), (b) *Whose child is it?* (e.g., we do not usurp families' decision-making role), and (c) *Caregivers are competent adults* (so we use adult-learning theory) (McWilliam, in preparation).

A third activity—and probably the most effective one—is parenting practices. Strength-based parenting has been found to have many benefits, both to children and caregivers (Waters, 2015). This approach involves caregivers' focusing on the positive attributes of the child and the family rather than on improving weaknesses. In early childhood intervention birth to 5 or 8 years, this can be challenging since, by definition, the child would have delays or disabilities making them eligible for services. But strength-based parenting might be especially important for these children to build their resilience, with self-esteem as a mediator, and to stave off learned helplessness (Loton & Waters, 2017). In one study, strength-based parenting predicted perseverance and engagement (Waters et al., 2019). In the RBM, persistence is in the highest level of engagement, therefore, practitioners should encourage families when they promote their children's perseverance/persistence.

Promoting resilience in children is vital, especially for children who face adverse conditions (Masten, 2018). Promoting resilience in caregivers is equally as important. The Surgeon General recently sent an advisory about the enormous stress parents are often under (Deater-Deckard, 1998; U.S. Surgeon General, 2024). Sometimes it is self-inflicted as they try to keep up with modern-day expectations for children's extracurricular activities, for always entertaining the child, and for enrolling the child in the best preschool. The situation is even more stressful for families of young children with disabilities, where families think they should get more and more services (Deater-Deckard, 1998), where the child might act out in the grocery store, or where the child's engagement in everyday routines is low (Weber, 2022). In the RBM, an ecomap is used to help assess the amount of support families receive from their informal support network and how much emotional support the caregivers receive within their family (McWilliam, 2010a).

Finally, the family is a source of resilience, by fostering emotional regulation and social competence through strong family relationships and caregiving as a buffer against stress (Walsh, 1996). Families are not homogeneous, so practitioners need to address the diverse needs of families (who will have different cultural and socioeconomic considerations) when helping families to have the capacity to be sources of resilience (Harry, 2002).

Facilitating Positive Functioning and Outcomes

The World Health Organization has produced the International Classification of Functioning, Disability and Health (ICF), a framework for coding the functioning of individuals to help organize supports and to monitor changes in a person's functioning (Leonardi et al., 2022). Two key elements of the ICF are the prominence of functioning, as opposed to IQ or simply diagnoses, and the relationship between functioning/disability and environmental factors. In the lives of young children, salient environmental factors are the ubiquitous presence of the family (usually) and other caregivers and the daily routines. We start with the role of the family.

Role of the Family

In the United States, the importance of "natural environments" is incorporated into the law establishing early intervention services (IDEA, 2004). This requirement has resulted in over 90% of families in early intervention receiving their services through home- and community-based (e.g., childcare) visits (U.S. Department of Education, 2017). The law does not, however, specify what the early intervention practitioner does once inside the home. In the RBM, one prevailing aphorism is *All the intervention occurs between visits*. This aphorism emphasizes two truths—that practitioners should help the *adults* in the family and that everyday routines ("activities" in the ICF) are the context in which intervention occurs.

In the same way that children who are typically developing learn through their daily routines, such as play, mealtimes, bath time, outside time, and so on, we believe it is an equity issue that children with disabilities should also learn in these typical times of the day. The role of early childhood intervention is to help families meet the unique needs of the child with specific strategies or adaptations. The cultural norms and preferences of the individual family are also important when working collaboratively to meet these needs (Garcia Grau et al., 2022).

What does this approach say about learning opportunities? Clearly, instead of one hour a week of one-on-one, hands-on intervention from a practitioner, the child now receives potentially hours of so-called intervention—and not from a relative stranger but from the child's regular caregiver (i.e., parent or other familiar figure) (Dunst, 2020). We use the term "so-called intervention" because it really is enhanced parenting. Caregivers are already teaching children in their many interactions with one another; in early childhood intervention, practitioners simply help them with that role.

Families' motivation for implementing interventions in their everyday life is often both their love for their child and their belief in the goals and the strategies. Goals (also referred to as outcomes) are what the team (theoretically) wants or expects the child to achieve in 6 months or a year. When goals are developed by practitioners, caregivers might not agree with them or understand them. Therefore, in the RBM, a method exists—the Routines-Based Interview (RBI)—that explores the child's functioning in home or classroom routines (Boavida et al., 2016). By asking for details about the child's engagement, independence, and social relationships, practitioners uncover many possibilities for goals. The RBI concludes with families' decisions on 10–12 goals for their child and family. This decision results in the family's having goals they care about and in their understanding that they are a crucial part of the decision-making process.

Following our earlier mention of natural environments, this mandate of the law is the equivalent of the school-age part of IDEA (i.e., Part B), where the mandate is for special education and related services to be provided in the least restrictive environment (IDEA, 2004). Both mandates address the concept of inclusion—that children should be enabled to learn in settings and ways that children without disabilities do. Excluding children from participating in the mainstream of society is considered dated and biased. The more severe the child's disabilities, including disruptive behavior, the harder inclusion might be, but it should always be a goal. In the RBM, this goal of inclusion focuses on methods at home, in childcare, and in school that promote the child's engagement (Hwang & Su, 2017). Engagement is at the heart of meaningful participation. As McWilliam et al. (1985) wrote 40 years ago, a child cannot learn if the child is not engaged.

Limitations of Current Knowledge

As scholars have noted, what we know about family-centered practice to date comes with some limitations. A call exists for improved understanding of practitioners' interpretations of family-centered practice to tailor training and support for professionals (Foster et al., 2020; Epley et al., 2010). Drawing on Romano and Schnurr's (2022) discussion of the research-to-practice divide specific to caregiver coaching and caregiver-implemented intervention, we acknowledge their principal divides: (a) Most research uses research staff to implement intervention rather than community-based practitioners, (b) a paucity of studies exists specific to training practitioners in their use of caregiver-implemented intervention approaches, (c) many studies focus on individual domains instead of using a primary service provider approach, (d) families' priorities might not align with the research package, and (e) family implementation of interventions is affected by intrafamily factors (Romano & Schnurr, 2022).

The solutions to these limitations and divides are obvious if not easy. They point to new approaches to research, especially implementation science (Fixsen et al., 2013; Romano & Schnurr, 2022). Researchers have more recently begun to conduct studies with consideration of the conditions described above (e.g., Rogers et al., 2022; Stahmer et al., 2020), however, additional work is needed to address more appropriately the present challenges and to support community uptake of evidence-based practice.

One of the major challenges in this line of research is the multiple steps involved in getting to child functioning, with parenting as a crucial step. Figure 7.1 shows this progression.

Future Directions

Given the complexities of family-centered practice, including caregiver-implemented intervention and caregiver coaching, early childhood practitioners and administrators might wonder where to go from here. One important step moving forward is evaluation of pre-service and in-service training to ensure stronger incorporation of

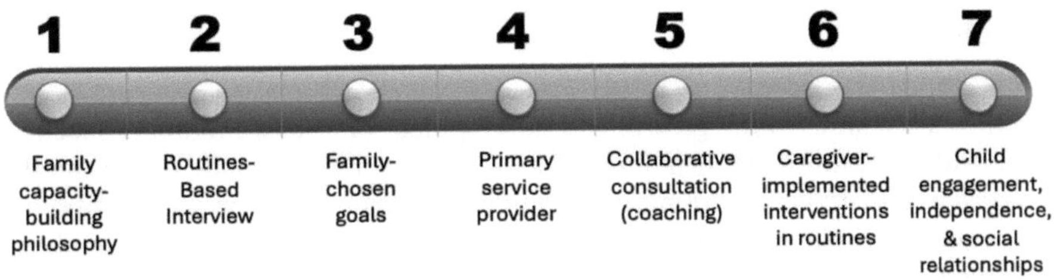

Fig. 7.1 Steps to child functioning

these practices into pre-service and in-service programs (Douglas et al., 2020; Gisewhite et al., 2021; Pellecchia et al., 2024). Although many topics often need to be covered in pre-service and in-service training, practitioners report that such training is insufficient to implement certain family-centered practices successfully (Douglas et al., 2020). Below, we describe some immediate steps practitioners can take to support their own use of family-centered practices when working with families of young children with disabilities and health conditions.

When a practitioner first begins working with a family, the initial phase of this collaborative partnership is crucial in setting the stage for services and establishing expectations for all involved parties. In the RBM, practitioners have a ground rules conversation with the family, describing the purpose of the visits and what the family can expect (McWilliam, 2010b). In other words, the practitioner provides a detailed description of everyone's roles, illustrating what the visits might look like (as well as what they will not look like). By doing this, practitioners can address the potential misperceptions families might have about services and make clarifications before getting started.

In addition, specific resources exist to support practitioners in assessing their level of family-centeredness when interacting with children and families. Table 7.3 provides a list of checklists available to evaluate one's family-centered practices. Continuous assessment and reflection of one's own practices is key to successful implementation of family-centered practices and to professional growth and development.

Table 7.3 Resources to promote family-centered practice

Resource	Website
ECTA Center Family Capacity-Building Checklist	https://ectacenter.org/~pdfs/decrp/FAM-4_Fam_Capacity-Building_2017.pdf
ECTA Center Family-Centered Practices Checklist	https://ectacenter.org/~pdfs/decrp/fam-1_fam-ctrd_practices_2017.pdf
ECTA Center Informed Family Decision-Making Practices Checklist	https://ectacenter.org/~pdfs/decrp/FAM-2_Inf_Family_Decision_2017.pdf
Checklist for Assessing Adherence to Family-Centered Practices	https://fipp.ncdhhs.gov/wp-content/uploads/casetools_vol1_no1.pdf

Conclusion

Families are central to the growth and development of young children, especially those with disabilities and health conditions. Research supports the use of family-centered practice when working with families of young children with disabilities and health conditions, and it is widely accepted and recommended across disciplines. Practitioners should evaluate how family centered they are when working with young children with disabilities and health conditions and consider ways they can build family capacity through evidence-based, family-centered practices to improve the lives of children and families.

References

Akemoglu, Y., & Meadan, H. (2018). Parent-implemented language and communication interventions for children with developmental delays and disabilities: A scoping review. *Review Journal of Autism and Developmental Disorders, 5*, 294–309. https://doi.org/10.1007/s40489-018-0140-x

Bailey, D. B., Buysse, V., Edmondson, R., & Smith, T. M. (1992). Creating family-centered services in early intervention: Perceptions of professionals in four states. *Exceptional Children, 58*(4), 298–309. https://doi.org/10.1177/001440299205800403

Bailey, D. B., Raspa, M., & Fox, L. C. (2012). What is the future of family outcomes and family-centered services? *Topics in Early Childhood Special Education, 31*(4), 216–223. https://doi.org/10.1177/0271121411427077

Barton, E. E., & Fettig, A. (2013). Parent-implemented interventions for young children with disabilities: A review of fidelity features. *Journal of Early Intervention, 35*(2), 194–219. https://doi.org/10.1177/1053815113504625

Boavida, T., Aguiar, C., McWilliam, R. A., & Correia, N. (2016). Effects of an in-service training program using the routines-based interview. *Topics in Early Childhood Special Education, 36*(2), 67–77. https://doi.org/10.1177/0271121415604327

Boavida, T., Silva, C., Aguiar, C., & McWilliam, R. A. (2022). Measuring professionals' perceptions about collaborative consultation in early childhood intervention. *International Journal of Inclusive Education, 26*(14), 1309–1326. https://doi.org/10.1080/13603116.2020.1806367

Bowen, M. (1966). The use of family theory in clinical practice. *Comprehensive Psychiatry, 7*, 345–374.

Bronfenbrenner, U. (1974). Developmental research, public policy, and the ecology of early childhood. *Child Development, 45*, 1–5.

Bruder, M. B., Catalino, T., Chiarello, L. A., Cox Mitchell, M., Deppe, J., Gundler, D., Kemp, P., LeMoine, S., Long, T., Muhlenhaupt, M., Prelock, P., Schefkind, S., Stayton, V., & Ziegler, D. (2019). Finding a common lens: Competencies across professional disciplines providing early childhood intervention. *Infants & Young Children, 32*(4), 280–293. https://doi.org/10.1097/IYC.0000000000000153

Campbell, P. H., & Sawyer, L. B. (2007). Supporting learning opportunities in natural settings through participation-based services. *Journal of Early Intervention, 29*(4), 287–305. https://doi.org/10.1177/105381510702900402

Campbell, P. H., & Sawyer, L. B. (2009). Changing early intervention providers' home visiting skills through participation in professional development. *Topics in Early Childhood Special Education, 28*(4), 219–234. https://doi.org/10.1177/0271121408328481

Cheng, W. M., Smith, T. B., Butler, M., Taylor, T. M., & Clayton, D. (2023). Effects of parent-implemented interventions on outcomes of children with autism: A meta-analysis. *Journal of Autism and Developmental Disorders, 2023, 53*, 4147–4163. https://doi.org/10.1007/s10803-022-05688-8

Crais, E. R., Roy, V. P., & Free, K. (2006). Parents' and professionals' perceptions of the implementation of family-centered practices in child assessments. *American Journal of Speech-Language Pathology, 15*(4), 365–377. https://doi.org/10.1044/1058-0360(2006/034)

Cunconan-Lahr, R., & Brotherson, M. J. (1996). Advocacy in disability policy: Parents and consumers as advocates. *Mental Retardation, 34*(6), 352–358.

Deater-Deckard, K. (1998). Parenting stress and child adjustment: Some old hypotheses and new questions. *Clinical Psychology: Science and Practice, 5*(3), 314–332. https://psycnet.apa.org/doi/10.1111/j.1468-2850.1998.tb00152.x

Division for Early Childhood. (2014). DEC recommended practices in early intervention/early childhood special education. http://www.dec-sped.org/recommendedpractices

Douglas, S. N., Meadan, H., & Kammes, R. (2020). Early interventionists' caregiver coaching: A mixed methods approach exploring experiences and practices. *Topics in Early Childhood Special Education, 40*(2), 84–96. https://doi.org/10.1177/0271121419829899

Dunst, C. (2002). Family-centered practices: Birth through high school. *The Journal of Special Education, 36*(3), 139–147. https://doi.org/10.1177/00224669020360030401

Dunst, C. J. (2020). Everyday learning opportunities of young children with and without developmental disabilities or delays. *International Journal of Early Childhood Environmental Education, 7*(3), 23–41.

Dunst, C. J., & Espe-Sherwindt, M. (2016). Family-centered practices in early childhood intervention. In B. Reichow, B. A. Boyd, E. E. Barton, & S. L. Odom (Eds.), *Handbook of early childhood special education* (pp. 37–55). Springer.

Dunst, C. J., & Trivette, C. M. (2009). Meta-analytic structural equation modeling of the influences of family-centered care on parent and child psychological health. *International Journal of Pediatrics, 2009*(1), 1–9. https://doi.org/10.1155/2009/576840

Dunst, C. J., & Trivette, C. M. (2014). Capacity-building family-systems intervention practices. In G. H. S. Singer, D. E. Biegel, & P. Conway (Eds.), *Family support and family caregiving across disabilities* (pp. 39–63). Routledge.

Dunst, C. J., Trivette, C. M., & Hamby, D. W. (2007). Meta-analysis of family-centered helpgiving practices research. *Mental Retardation and Developmental Disabilities Research Reviews, 13*(4), 370–378. https://doi.org/10.1002/mrdd.20176

Epley, P., Gotto, G. S., Summers, J. A., Brotherson, M. J., Turnbull, A. P., & Friend, A. (2010). Supporting families of young children with disabilities: Examining the role of administrative structures. *Topics in Early Childhood Special Education, 30*(1), 20–31. https://doi.org/10.1177/0271121410363400

Fixsen, D., Blasé, K., Metz, A., & Van Dyke, M. (2013). Statewide implementation of evidence-based programs. *Exceptional Children, 79*(3), 213–230. https://doi.org/10.1177/001440291307900206

Foster, T. D., Decker, K. B., Vaterlaus, M., & Belleville, A. (2020). How early intervention practitioners described family-centred practice: A collective broadening of the definition. *Child: Care, Health, and Development, 46*(3), 268–274. https://doi.org/10.1111/cch.12749

Friedman, M., Woods, J., & Salisbury, C. (2012). Caregiver coaching strategies for early intervention providers: Moving toward operational definitions. *Infants & Young Children, 25*(1), 62–82. https://doi.org/10.1097/IYC.0b013e31823d8f12

Garcia Grau, P., Pedernera García, M. A., Barranco, S., McWilliam, R. A., & Morales Murillo, C. (2022). Modelo Basado en Rutinas y diversidad familiar, social y cultural. Cinco escenarios de acercamiento a las familias. In M. Frugone-Jaramillo & M. Gràcia (Eds.), *Hacia la adopción de prácticas centradas en la familia en América Latina: Primeras experiencias y aprendizajes* (pp. 23–55). Colección Case Grande.

García-Ventura, S., Mas, J. M., Balcells-Balcells, A., & Giné, C. (2021). Family-centred early intervention: Comparing practitioners' actual and desired practices. *Child: Care, Health, and Development, 47*(2), 218–227. https://doi.org/10.1111/cch.12834

Gisewhite, R. A., Jeanfreau, M. M., & Holden, C. L. (2021). A call for ecologically based teacher-parent communication skills training in pre-service teacher education programmes. *Educational Review, 73*(5), 597–616. https://doi.org/10.1080/00131911.2019.1666794

Green, J., Charman, T., McConachie, H., Aldred, C., Slonims, V., Howlin, P., Le Couteur, A., Leadbitter, K., Hudry, K., Byford, S., Barrett, B., Temple, K., Macdonald, W., & Pickles, A. (2010). Parent-mediated communication-focused treatment in children with autism (PACT): A randomised controlled trial. *The Lancet, 375*(9732), 2152–2160. https://doi.org/10.1016/S0140-6736(10)60587-9

Griffith, S. F., Magariño, L. S., Martínez Pedraza, F. D., Frazier, S. L., Berkovits, M. D., & Bagner, D. M. (2023). Surveying early intervention providers to identify opportunities for workforce support to strengthen family-centered care. *Infants & Young Children, 36*(4), 314–332. https://doi.org/10.1097/IYC.0000000000000247

Harry, B. (2002). Trends and issues in serving culturally diverse families of children with disabilities. *The Journal of Special Education, 36*(3), 131–138. https://doi.org/10.1177/00224669020360030301

Heidlage, J. K., Cunningham, J. E., Kaiser, A. P., Trivette, C. M., Barton, E. B., Frey, J. R., & Roberts, M. Y. (2020). The effects of parent-implemented language interventions on child linguistic outcomes: A meta-analysis. *Early Childhood Research Quarterly, 50*(1), 6–23. https://doi.org/10.1016/j.ecresq.2018.12.006

Hwang, A.-W., & Su, H.-C. (2017, November 16–17). *The preschool engagement intervention in Taiwan,* Engagement in Young children working conference for researchers, Jönköping University.

Individuals with Disabilities Education Improvement Act (IDEA) of 2004, 20 U.S.C. § 1400 (2004).

Kasari, C., Lawton, K., Shih, W., Barker, T. V., Landa, R., Lord, C., Orlich, F., King, B., Wetherby, A., & Senturk, D. (2014). Caregiver-mediated intervention for low-resourced preschoolers with autism: An RCT. *Pediatrics, 134*(1), e72–e79. https://doi.org/10.1542/peds.2013-3229

Kemp, P., & Turnbull, A. P. (2014). Coaching with parents in early intervention an interdisciplinary research synthesis. *Infants and Young Children, 27*(4), 305–324. https://doi.org/10.1097/IYC.0000000000000018

Kim, G. Y., Tuck, K. N., Eddy, M. M., Bhattashali, A., & Bigelow, K. M. (2025). Caregivers' perceptions on caregiver-implemented intervention and coaching. *Early Childhood Research Quarterly, 70*(1), 264–273. https://doi.org/10.1016/j.ecresq.2024.10.009

Kuhlthau, K. A., Bloom, S., Van Cleave, J., Knapp, A. A., Romm, D., Klatka, K., Homer, C. J., Newacheck, P. W., & Perrin, J. M. (2011). Evidence for family-centered care for children with special health care needs: A systematic review. *Academic Pediatrics, 11*(2), 136–143. https://doi.org/10.1016/j.acap.2010.12.014

Leonardi, M., Lee, H., Kostanjsek, N., Fornari, A., Raggi, A., Martinuzzi, A., Yáñez, M., Almborg, A.-H., Fresk, M., Besstrashnova, Y., et al. (2022). 20 years of ICF—International classification of functioning, disability and health: Uses and applications around the world. *International Journal of Environmental Research and Public Health, 19*(18), 11321. https://doi.org/10.3390/ijerph191811321

Loton, D. J., & Waters, L. E. (2017). The mediating effect of self-efficacy in the connections between strength-based parenting, happiness and psychological distress in teens. *Frontiers in Psychology, 8*, 1–13. https://doi.org/10.3389/fpsyg.2017.01707

Masten, A. S. (2018). Resilience theory and research on children and families: Past, present, and promise. *Journal of Family Theory & Review, 10*(1), 12–31. https://doi.org/10.1111/jftr.12255

McBroom, L. A., & Enriquez, M. (2009). Review of family-centered interventions to enhance the health outcomes of children with type 1 diabetes. *The Diabetes Educator, 35*(3), 428–438. https://doi.org/10.1177/0145721709332814

McWilliam, R. A. (2000). It's only natural… to have early intervention in the environments where it's needed. In S. Sandall & M. Ostrosky (Eds.), *Young exceptional children monograph series no. 2: Natural environments and inclusion* (pp. 17–26). The Division for Early Childhood of the Council for Exceptional Children.

McWilliam, R. A. (2010a). *Routines-based early intervention: Supporting young children with special needs and their families*. Paul H. Brookes.

McWilliam, R. A. (Ed.). (2010b). *Working with families of young children with special needs*. Guilford Press.

McWilliam, R. A. (2012). Implementing and preparing for home visits. *Topics in Early Childhood Special Education, 31*(4), 224–231. https://doi.org/10.1177/0271121411426488

McWilliam, R. A. (2016). Metanoia in early intervention: Transformation to a family-centered approach. *Revista Latinoamericana de Educación Inclusiva, 10*(1), 155–173.

McWilliam, R. A. (in preparation). *Aphorisms for early childhood interventionists to live by*.

McWilliam, R. A., & Scott, S. (2001). A support approach to early intervention: A three-part framework. *Infants & Young Children, 13*(4), 55–62.

McWilliam, R. A., Trivette, C. M., & Dunst, C. J. (1985). Behavior engagement as a measure of the efficacy of early intervention. *Analysis and Intervention in Developmental Disabilities, 5*(1–2), 59–71. https://doi.org/10.1016/S0270-4684(85)80006-9

Movahedazarhouligh, S. (2021). Parent-implemented interventions and family-centered service delivery approaches in early intervention and early childhood special education. *Early Child Development and Care, 191*(1), 1–12. https://doi.org/10.1080/03004430.2019.1603148

Movahedazarhouligh, S., & Banerjee, R. (2020). Leadership in implementation of quality family-centred services in early childhood: An exploration of administrators' perceptions, needs, and realities. *Early Child Development and Care, 190*(6), 948–962. https://doi.org/10.1080/03004430.2018.1503256

National Association for the Education of Young Children. (2020). *Developmentally appropriate practice in early childhood programs serving children from birth through age 8 (Position statement)*. https://www.naeyc.org/sites/default/files/globally-shared/downloads/PDFs/resources/position-statements/dap-statement_0.pdf

Pellecchia, M., Maye, M., Tomczuk, L., Zhong, N., Mandell, D. S., & Stahmer, A. C. (2024). Brief report: A scoping review of caregiver coaching strategies within caregiver-mediated interventions for autism. *Infants & Young Children, 37*(4), 336–350. https://doi.org/10.1097/IYC.0000000000000276

Peterson, C. A., Luze, G. J., Eshbaugh, E. M., Jeon, H. J., & Kantz, K. R. (2007). Enhancing parent-child interactions through home visiting: Promising practice or unfulfilled promise? *Journal of Early Intervention, 29*(2), 119–140. https://doi.org/10.1177/105381510702900205

Rieth, S. R., Stahmer, A. C., & Brookman-Frazee, L. (2018). A community collaborative approach to scaling-up evidence-based practices: Moving parent-implemented interventions from research to practice. In M. Siller & L. Morgan (Eds.), *Handbook of parent-implemented interventions for very young children with autism* (pp. 441–458). Springer.

Roberts, M. Y., & Kaiser, A. P. (2011). The effectiveness of parent-implemented language interventions: A meta-analysis. *American Journal of Speech-Language Pathology, 20*(3), 180–199. https://doi.org/10.1044/1058-0360(2011/10-0055)

Rogers, S. J., Estes, A., Lord, C., Vismara, L., Winter, J., Fitzpatrick, A., Guo, M., & Dawson, G. (2012). Effects of a brief Early Start Denver Model (ESDM)-based parent intervention on toddlers at risk for autism spectrum disorders: A randomized controlled trial. *Journal of the American Academy of Child & Adolescent Psychiatry, 51*(10), 1052–1065. https://doi.org/10.1016/j.jaac.2012.08.003

Rogers, S. J., Vismara, L. A., & Dawson, G. (2021). *Coaching parents of young children with autism: Promoting connection, communication, and learning*. The Guildford Press.

Rogers, S. J., Stahmer, A., Talbott, M., Young, G., Fuller, E., Pellecchia, M., Barber, A., & Griffith, E. (2022). Feasibility of delivering parent-implemented NDBI interventions in low-resource regions: A pilot randomized controlled study. *Journal of Neurodevelopmental Disorders, 14*(3), 1–14. https://doi.org/10.1186/s11689-021-09410-0

Romano, M., & Schnurr, M. (2022). Mind the gap: Strategies to bridge the research-to-pratice divide in early intervention caregiver coaching practices. *Topics in Early Childhood Special Education, 42*(1), 64–76. https://doi.org/10.1177/0271121419899163

Romano, M., Lorio, C., Delehanty, A., Eugenio, J., Abarca, D., Trivedi, B., & Brown, J. A. (2022). Family routines within caregiver-implemented early interventions: A scoping review. *Journal of Early Intervention, 44*(4), 371–392. https://doi.org/10.1177/10538151211062206

Rush, D. D., & Shelden, M. L. (2019). *The early childhood coaching handbook* (2nd ed.). Paul H. Brookes.

Sawyer, B. E., & Campbell, P. H. (2017). Teaching caregivers in early intervention. *Infants & Young Children, 30*(3), 175–189. https://doi.org/10.1097/IYC.0000000000000094

Shelden, M. L., & Rush, D. D. (2022). *The early intervention teaming handbook: The primary service provider approach* (2nd edition). Paul H. Brookes.

Stadnick, N. A., Stahmer, A., & Brookman-Frazee, L. (2015). Preliminary effectiveness of Project ImPACT: A parent-mediated intervention for children with autism spectrum disorder delivered in a community program. *Journal of Autism and Developmental Disorders, 45*, 2092–2104. https://doi.org/10.1007/s10803-015-2376-y

Stahmer, A. C., Rieth, S. R., Dickson, K. S., Feder, J., Burgeson, M., Searcy, K., & Brookman-Frazee, L. (2020). Project ImPACT for toddlers: Pilot outcomes of a community adaptation of an intervention for autism risk. *Autism, 24*(3), 617–632. https://doi.org/10.1177/1362361319878080

Stein, R., Steed, E., & Charlifue-Smith, R. (2025). Professionals' reported practices to involve families in initial evaluations for early intervention and early childhood special education: A mixed methods study. *Infants & Young Children, 38*(1), 22–39. https://doi.org/10.1097/IYC.0000000000000280

Swanson, J., Raab, M., & Dunst, C. J. (2011). Strengthening family capacity to provide young children everyday natural learning opportunities. *Journal of Early Childhood Research, 9*(1), 66–80. https://doi.org/10.1177/1476718X10368588

Tomeny, K. R., McWilliam, R. A., & Tomeny, T. S. (2020). Caregiver-implemented intervention for young children with autism spectrum disorder: A systematic review of coaching components. *Review Journal of Autism and Developmental Disorders, 7*, 168–181. https://doi.org/10.1007/s40489-019-00186-7

Tomeny, K. R., García-Grau, P., & McWilliam, R. A. (2021). Early interventionists' ratings of family-centered practices in natural environments. *Infants & Young Children, 34*, 266–283. https://doi.org/10.1097/IYC.0000000000000203

Trivette, C. M., Dunst, C. J., Hamby, D. W., & O'Herin, C. E. (2009). Characteristics and consequences of adult learning methods and strategies. *Research Brief, 3*, 1–33.

U.S. Department of Education. (2017). *39th annual report to congress on the implementation of the Individuals with Disabilities Education Act*. Office of Special Education and Rehabilitative Services.

U.S. Surgeon General. (2024). *Under pressure: U.S. Surgeon General's advisory on the mental health & well-being of parents*. Washington, DC.

Walsh, F. (1996). The concept of family resilience: Crisis and challenge. *Family Process, 35*(3), 261–281. https://doi.org/10.1111/j.1545-5300.1996.00261.x

Waters, L. (2015). The relationship between strength-based parenting with children's stress levels and strength-based coping approaches. *Psychology, 6*(6), 689. https://doi.org/10.4236/psych.2015.66067

Waters, L. E., Loton, D., & Jach, H. K. (2019). Does strength-based parenting predict academic achievement? The mediating effects of perseverance and engagement. *Journal of Happiness Studies, 20*, 1121–1140. https://doi.org/10.1007/s10902-018-9983-1

Weber, E. T. (2022). Stoic pragmatism for parenting a child with disabilities: An essay addressing philosophers, parents, teachers, and educational policymakers. In N. Whelan-Jackson & D. J. Brunson (Eds.), *Disability and American philosophies* (pp. 182–198). Routledge.

Windsor, K. S., Woods, J., Kaiser, A. P., Snyder, P., & Salisbury, C. (2019). Caregiver-implemented intervention for communication and motor outcomes for infants and toddlers. *Topics in Early Childhood Special Education, 39*(2), 73–87. https://doi.org/10.1177/0271121418815250

Wong, C., Odom, S. L., Hume, K. A., Cox, A. W., Fettig, A., Kucharczyk, S., Brock, M. E., Plavnick, J. B., Fleury, V. P., & Schultz, T. R. (2015). Evidence-based practices for children, youth, and young adults with autism spectrum disorder: A comprehensive review. *Journal for Autism and Developmental Disorders, 45*, 1951–1966. https://doi.org/10.1007/s10803-014-2351-z

Woods, J. (2024). Family guided routines based intervention. https://fgrbi.com/

Woods, J. J., Wilcox, M. J., Friedman, M., & Murch, T. (2011). Collaborative consultation in natural environments: Strategies to enhance family-centered supports and services. *Language, Speech, and Hearing Services in Schools, 42*(3), 379–392. https://doi.org/10.1044/0161-1461(2011/10-0016)

Chapter 8
Peer Support and Resilience for Young Children with Medical Conditions or Neurodiversity

Isabella K. Pallotto, Francesca A. St. Pe, Taylor Gates, Harrison Powers, and Cathleen Odar Stough

Abstract This chapter examines how peer support contributes to resilience, inclusion, and social development for young children with medical conditions or neurodiversity. Peer-mediated interventions, such as buddy systems, effectively build prosocial behaviors, foster friendships, and promote environments where children with and without disabilities can thrive. Peers, typically children with strong social skills and consistent attendance, act as partners and role models, creating natural opportunities for communication, play, and social learning. The chapter emphasizes that peer support benefits both children with medical conditions or neurodiversity and the peer supporters themselves, increasing empathy, reducing stigma, and boosting sensitivity to diversity. It discusses summer camps and peer-based activities as important contexts for social connection and self-confidence. The chapter also identifies a research gap, as most studies target adolescents rather than younger children. Overall, it argues that well-designed peer support can enhance quality of life and inclusion for children with diverse needs, but further research on early interventions is needed.

Keywords Children with developmental disabilities · Peer-mediated interventions · Supports for peer interventions · Social skill development · Peer support · Social isolation · Neurodiversity · Interventions for peer support

Peer support is a reciprocal relationship of giving and receiving help with someone with shared experiences and similar identities (Shalaby & Agyapong, 2020). For young children with a medical condition or who experience neurodiversity, peer support, often provided through peer-mediated interventions (PMIs) (Devine et al., 2016; Reichow & Song, 2024), may enhance relationships and connection with peers without developmental or health conditions (i.e., medical conditions or neurodiversity). Inclusion and peer support from typically developing and healthy peers has

I. K. Pallotto · F. A. St. Pe · T. Gates · H. Powers · C. O. Stough (✉)
Department of Psychology, University of Cincinnati, Cincinnati, OH, USA
e-mail: odarcc@ucmail.uc.edu

L. Nabors and T. Stanton-Chapman (eds.), *Developmental Disabilities and Chronic Illness in Young Children*, Springer Series on Child and Family Studies,
https://doi.org/10.1007/978-3-032-08523-8_8

numerous benefits for children with medical conditions or who experience neurodiversity, including promoting positive development (e.g., social, moral, language and cognitive), overall health and wellbeing, resilience, belonging, and quality of life (Coleman et al., 2017; Graham, 2023; Parker et al., 2015; Stewart & Sun, 2004; Uslu & Gizir, 2017). Peer support offers both psychological (e.g., emotional support) and material resources (e.g., sharing of information, assistance with tasks) that can promote positive emotions, self-worth, predictability, self-esteem, and self-efficacy (Chu et al., 2010; Coleman et al., 2017). Inclusion may be particularly important for children who have been demonstrated to be at-risk for social exclusion, particularly for those with emotional, behavioral, or developmental disabilities or severe impairment (Koller et al., 2018). Early intervention during young childhood can play a critical role in supporting social development and social inclusion later in childhood (Koller et al., 2018).

The current chapter examines the benefits and need for peer interaction and support among young children (3–8 years) with medical conditions or who experience neurodiversity. The research we review highlights the benefits of peer support and unique considerations for peer support for young children with a range of medical and neurodevelopmental conditions. Further, interventions promoting positive peer relationships and social inclusion (e.g., PMIs) are reviewed. Lastly, clinical implications and practical applications are discussed as well as future directions for research, policy, and practice.

The Importance of Peers for Young Children

The social and peer landscape evolves significantly throughout early life and the primary school years. Peer relationships begin to develop as early as infancy and toddlerhood with children placing increased attention on peer relationships starting in their preschool years (Parker et al., 2015). Peer involvement increases to represent a large portion of social interaction for children by middle school (Gifford-Smith & Brownell, 2003; Parker et al., 2015). Young childhood represents a significant developmental period for children, and early childhood is an essential stage for developing socioemotional skills like conflict resolution, emotion regulation, and problem solving (Willard et al., 2021; Woodhead et al., 1999). During this developmental period, young children establish an increased understanding of social settings, early social skills, and socialization through increased social interaction (Malik & Marwaha, 2022). At this age, children build social relationships and social skills that will be used for developing future social relationships as they age (Rubin & Ross, 2012). Establishing these relationships and skills before the onset of puberty is important given increases in peer exclusion that happen during puberty (Carter et al., 2018). Social skills development of young children also includes expanding skills for use across multiple social settings (e.g., preschool or elementary school) and developing distinct relationships in different areas of social life (e.g., family, friends, classmates; Webster-Stratton & Reid, 2004). For example, engaging in social interactions with similarly aged peers in a school environment involves a separate set of social skills and norms for interaction than social interactions with family and adults. Peer interactions and peer support can offer the opportunity for developing these important social skills at a young age.

Family and environmental support are significant contributors to peer support. Families play a significant role in facilitating early peer relationships, especially because they establish the settings wherein peer relationships are often created (Lamb & Bornstein, 2013). For example, parents typically determine or guide the home environment, interactions with extended family and involvement in extracurricular activities and religious settings, which are places where early childhood relationships are established. Adults in the child's environment can also assist in fostering social inclusion by structuring and providing opportunities for children to socialize and be exposed to social environments or interactions. Allowing young children opportunities to build confidence through independent social interactions is also important with caregivers providing guidance as appropriate on navigating these newfound relationships with peers (e.g., providing guidance on social reciprocity, instruction and modeling regarding social behaviors that are appropriate in various settings). One of the primary settings in which peer interactions and social support occur is early childcare settings, where children can develop relationships with caregivers beyond the family (i.e., with teachers) and relationships with peers in a group environment. Early childcare and school environments are also an effective avenue for implementation of peer support systems (Baginsky, 2004).

Peer Support for Children with Medical Conditions and Neurodivergence Disabilities

Peers can provide considerable psychosocial support to children with a medical condition or who experience neurodiversity (e.g., children with autism spectrum disorder; ASD). While research regarding social support is often focused on adolescents, limited research has demonstrated that social support is a protective factor in adapting to and coping with a medical condition or neurodivergence specifically among young children (Brown, 2004; Van Der Laan et al., 2023). Evidence has shown that the development of peer relationships and peer support for neurodivergent youth or youth with medical conditions is a crucial part of a child's social and emotional development, fostering social skills and good mental health (La Greca et al., 2002; Van Der Laan et al., 2023). Many medical conditions co-occur with psychological disorders (e.g., anxiety, depression) and/or neurodevelopmental conditions (e.g., ASD, attention-deficit hyperactivity disorder, ADHD; Johnson et al., 2021). For older children experiencing medical conditions or neurodivergence, strong friendships are protective against anxiety and depression (La Greca & Harrison, 2005; Van Harmelen et al., 2016), which may be similarly protective for young children.

The wellbeing of children with medical conditions or neurodiversity appears to be linked to peer inclusion. Friendships and social support can facilitate children's adjustment to a diagnosis (Brown, 2004). Strong friend and family support at times of diagnosis are associated with fewer externalizing and internalizing symptoms (Brown, 2004). Peer support can also help improve health–related quality of life for children, and research has consistently highlighted the importance of continuing and prioritizing peer socialization during treatment (af Sandeberg et al., 2008; McLoone et al., 2013; Plage et al., 2022). Peer support also is related to positive social development, and it also mitigates the isolation that children can experience as they cope with medical regimens, appointments, and therapies related to their conditions (McLoone et al., 2013; Plage et al., 2022).

Social Isolation

The isolation children with medical conditions or neurodiversity face may hinder abilities to make and keep friends. Research results are equivocal as to whether children with medical conditions display differences in social skills compared to children without these conditions (Darcy et al., 2014, 2019; Fraser, 2003; Martinez et al., 2011; McLoone et al., 2013; Nassau & Drotar, 1995; Noll et al., 2010; Tse et al., 2007; Willard et al., 2021). However, there are risk factors related to the social functioning of children with medical conditions. For example, children with medical conditions that impact their physical or cognitive development commonly express difficulties with emotion regulation, communication, and prosocial behaviors, contributing to struggles to follow rules and expectations, increasing their likelihood of being isolated, suspended, and expelled from school settings (Harjusola-Webb et al., 2012; Petry & Maes, 2007). Moreover, research has shown that children with medical conditions that impact their physical or cognitive development commonly express difficulties with emotion regulation, communication, and prosocial behaviors, contributing to struggles to follow rules and expectations, increasing their likelihood of being isolated, suspended, and expelled from school settings (Harjusola-Webb et al., 2012; Petry & Maes, 2007).

Evidence is clearer for neurodivergent children, specifically children with ASD (Baron-Cohen et al., 1985). Some neurodiverse children may engage in challenging behaviors (e.g., aggression, destruction, tantrums, shutting down) that distance them from their peers (Chang & Locke, 2016). Risks may be more pronounced for some children with ASD. For instance, young children with ASD have been shown to have fewer reciprocal friendships, smaller social networks, and be more disengaged with peers on the playground compared to children without ASD (Chang & Locke, 2016). Support or activity groups where children can establish relationships with peers with parallel or similar challenges could remove many barriers to making friends for these young children.

There are some commonalities related to risk for social interactions for children with either developmental or medical conditions. Those with conditions that impact their physical or cognitive development commonly express difficulties with emotion regulation, communication, and prosocial behaviors, contributing to struggles to follow rules and expectations, increasing their likelihood of being isolated, suspended, and expelled from school settings (Harjusola-Webb et al., 2012; Petry & Maes, 2007). Also, children with major limitations (e.g., self-injurious behavior, quadriplegia, cognitive impairment, airway clearance) due to neurodivergence or a medical condition may spend less time with peers and engage in fewer social activities (Kuutti et al., 2022). Children with complex communication needs *and* physical disability may also have less frequent social interactions, engage with a fewer number of peers, and engage in a smaller variety of activities compared to matched, typically developing peers (Thirumanickam et al., 2011). Research focusing on the impact of comorbid conditions is less common, and will provide information to guide the field.

Overcoming Low Levels of Support

Clinicians and medical professionals should assess the extent of peer support needs and socialization. Red flags may include lack of participation in extracurricular activities, recess, or "specials" (e.g., physical education class) because of the activities' lack of accessibility or physical demands (Johnson et al., 2021). For example, during this age period, children often engage with peers through extracurricular physical activities (e.g., ballet, soccer, tee ball, gymnastics), and, oftentimes, these activities are not inclusive to children with medical conditions who require assistive devices (e.g., wheelchairs, braces, or canes) or to children who are neurodivergent and may require modifications to understand and become involved in activities. Ensuring that the medical team meets with staff and teaches them about child needs and abilities, and ways to involve the child in activities may improve inclusion. Many times, these activities are not adaptive because staff are not trained in how to safely integrate the child with a medical condition (Johnson et al., 2021).

Additionally, parents of children with medical conditions, such as epilepsy, may limit their child's engagement in activities due to safety concerns, even if medical staff feel it is safe for their child to participate (Johnson et al., 2021). Meetings with parents and the medical team may help parents implement accommodations to involve their children in these activities. Alternately, referral to counseling may be helpful in allowing parents to share concerns and brainstorm ideas for increasing their children's involvement in different types of activities with peers. Similarly, children with complex medical conditions may have relatively fewer opportunities to connect with same-age peers because of communication challenges and increased time spent with paid workers such as caretakers or members of the hospital team (Nijs et al., 2016; Thirumanickam et al., 2011). Meetings with school staff and the medical team should address communication challenges and referral for speech therapy or meetings with the school staff to include counseling as part of educational planning may provide the coaching children need to improve pragmatic language skills or social communication.

Missing School Opportunities

Absenteeism among children with medical conditions may also negatively impact opportunities for social support because it can cause social isolation from peers. Children with medical conditions have higher absenteeism from school than healthy children because of doctor's appointments, inpatient hospitalizations, and fatigue associated with their conditions (af Sandeberg et al., 2008; Barker & Quittner, 2016; Darcy et al., 2019; Pawlowski et al., 2019; Willard et al., 2021). Additionally, children with congenital medical conditions, such as cystic fibrosis, may also have more consistent absenteeism because of constant disease management responsibilities (Barker & Quittner, 2016). Children with medical conditions who are immunocompromised are also often required to be absent for infection control purposes, particularly during cold and flu season or during an illness flare (Barker & Quittner, 2016; McLoone et al., 2013).

Absenteeism from school due to health is associated with decreased health-related quality of life in children with a medical condition (af Sandeberg et al., 2008; McLoone et al., 2013). School re-entry (returning to school after an inpatient hospitalization) is a key moment for supporting the inclusion of children with medical conditions. When returning to school, these children may be less confident when interacting with peers, often not knowing how to engage with their classmates (McLoone et al., 2013). These children also demonstrated considerable anxiety about participating in activities that they previously were not allowed to do due to risk for infection (e.g., playing in the sandbox) and experienced difficulties with turn-taking (McLoone et al., 2013). However, at this age, parents can build resilience in children's social development. For young children, social skills are often developed through interactions with the family, particularly through interactions with parents and siblings (Hoyne & Egan, 2024). Thus, even if a child with a medical condition misses out on social experiences outside of the home, they can still develop social skills with members of the family unit (Hoyne & Egan, 2024).

Further research is needed to more broadly understand social skills development among children with medical conditions or neurodiversity. Results are mixed on whether children with medical conditions display differences in social skills (Martinez et al., 2011; Tse et al., 2007). Several studies found no difference in social competence between children with a medical condition and healthy children and between children with different medical conditions (Nassau & Drotar, 1995; Noll et al., 2010). However, other authors argue that due to increased social isolation, children with medical conditions at this age fail to develop social skills comparable to healthy peers (Darcy et al., 2014, 2019; Fraser, 2003; McLoone et al., 2013; Tse et al., 2007; Willard et al., 2021). At this age, social skills are often developed through interactions with the family, particularly through interactions with parents and siblings. Thus, even if a child with a medical condition misses out on social experiences outside of the home, they can still develop social skills with members of the family unit. The evidence for challenges with social skills is clearer for neurodivergent children. Difficulty with social skills is a hallmark of ASD (Baron-Cohen et al., 1985). Young children with ASD have been shown to have fewer reciprocal friendships, smaller social networks, and be more unengaged with peers on the playground compared to children without ASD (Chang & Locke, 2016). Current research suggests that children with medical conditions or neurodiversity would benefit from interventions to improve social skills.

Improving Peer Support for Children with Medical Conditions and Children with Neurodiversity

The role of interventions, specifically ones that utilize peer support, have been successful in addressing needs for inclusivity, and have been effective in increasing prosocial behaviors and positive interactions among children with and without medical conditions or neurodiversity (Harjusola-Webb et al., 2012). Peers are typically children without conditions or disabilities but are defined differently across peer-involved interventions; children who are nominated to be a peer (e.g., peer buddy) are most often similar in age and grade as the child needing support, and who have regular attendance, appropriate social skills, and a high social status in the classroom (Chang & Locke, 2016). However, peers do not necessarily need to be "typically developing" or "healthy;" children can learn from peers who share similarities in experience through having a shared condition, including those with similar diagnoses or those who have acquired proficiency in a specific skill or behavior. If a peer "buddy" is enthusiastic about interacting with others and has good social skills, this can facilitate support and social interaction for a child with a medical condition or neurodiversity (Gunning et al., 2019).

Peers can serve as playmates or communication partners (Hanline et al., 2022), creating a natural setting for children who struggle to maintain social interactions or friendships to learn and practice social skills. Research has also shown that peers themselves also benefit from these interventions; child peers experience increased positive interactions with children of differing abilities and increased sensitivity to others with an increase in knowledge about different medical or neurodevelopmental conditions and disabilities (Gunning et al., 2019), which can further decrease stigmatization of children with disabilities or conditions and increase the quality of social support, connections, and friendships.

Summer Camps

There are various types of interventions and related methods that utilize peers to support children with medical conditions and neurodiversity. Peers have successfully been leveraged in interventions taking place in various settings, like camps. Summer camp program interventions for children (and their families) have been shown to improve mood, self-concept, empathy, and emotional wellbeing; these factors are related to positive interactions with others (Christiansen et al., 2015; Martiniuk et al., 2014). Additionally, participation in camps, where children with similar conditions receive support and interact with each other, has been associated with improved friendships and decreased isolation (Christiansen et al., 2015; Martiniuk et al., 2014). Summer programs for children often positively impact illness-related knowledge (Martiniuk et al., 2014). Increased knowledge about one's condition and abilities can improve children's confidence and abilities to engage in activities with their peers. Among older children, camp attendance has been associated with slight improvements in self-perception (i.e., self-esteem, self-concept; Odar et al., 2013), which may have broader implications on how children interact with others and their friendships with peers. For younger children, family and sibling day camps afford opportunities to receive peer support and participate in positive interactions; learning how to engage in sports and activities provide participation experience that is applicable to other settings like afterschool and community activities.

Interventions in Educational Settings

Like summer camps, involving peers in academic settings has also been shown to be effective (Van Der Meulen et al., 2021). Evidence supports that educating children with health conditions or neurodiversity alongside typically developing peers allows for increased access to learning opportunities, accommodations, and systems-level support (National Association for the Education of & Young Children & Division for Early Childhood., 2009). Peers in academic settings can help address low grades or learning deficits due to school absenteeism, aid with the school re-entry transition, and increase children's interactions with student peers. Parents and caregivers can also request intervention from school counselors, teachers, and leaders of extracurricular activities to help involve their child with peers. Meetings with a treatment team can provide education to these professionals to facilitate plans for social involvement that can be optimized to meet child needs (Plage et al., 2022). Since the COVID-19 pandemic, virtual learning and social opportunities have been accessible in more formats (e.g., telehealth), making team meetings more of a possibility, as key players can meet online rather than having to travel between locations, such as schools and clinics. Counselors can also work with children through telehealth to build skills for group entry and interacting with peers. However, learning in a virtual environment can be challenging for young children with medical conditions or neurodiversity, and finding ways to model and practice skills "online," in a developmentally appropriate way for young children, remains an area for future research (Ford et al., 2021). More research in this area is needed to understand and expand the capacities of virtual learning for this population, particularly in supporting the development of positive peer relationships among younger children.

Interventions Focusing on Peers

Peer interventions also focus on emotional support, via methods like befriending, mediation or conflict resolution, and counseling-based approaches (Van Der Meulen et al., 2021). Befriending can resemble companionship among children with medical conditions or neurodiversity and peers to alleviate bullying and solitude and address difficulties making friends. Conflict resolution can address strategies for resolving disagreements between peers or adults, which may be common among children who have externalizing behaviors and subsequent difficulties with social interactions. Counseling-based interventions may aid in teaching listening and communication skills and empathy for children who may exhibit social or emotional difficulties. The effectiveness of an emotion-support peer intervention has been shown to address emotional relief and self-esteem and increase children's abilities to cope with problems and communication skills (Van Der Meulen et al., 2021).

Peers have also been included in psychosocial treatment approaches to address social deficits that may interfere with children's abilities to develop and maintain social relationships with others their age and grade. Most commonly, these are implemented in school systems where children interact with others their age. These approaches are referred to as peer involvement, peer proximity, and peer mediation (Van Der Meulen et al., 2021). Peer involvement utilizes children aiding each other's learning to practice social skills. Peer proximity refers to when a child needing more support is seated near another child who models skills necessary for appropriate social interactions.

Peer Mediated Interventions (PMIs) encompass a broad class of evidence-based interventions (e.g., buddy skills, integrated play, peer-mediated social interaction training) in which peers are systematically trained to engage in positive social interactions through an instructional role to support the development of a specific skill, primarily, among children with neurodiversity (Odom & Strain, 1984). PMIs are effective across a variety of settings for children, such as school classrooms, playgrounds, and homes (Reichow & Song, 2024) with most being focused on improving support in structured classroom settings. Additionally, as children age and enter preschool or elementary school, the involvement of peers can allow for increased support as children's dependence on their family decreases over time (Kazemi et al., 2016). PMI procedures can be carried out during structured times, like recess or playtime, lasting between 10 and 15 min to naturally incorporate increased opportunities for social interactions and skills development (Gunning et al., 2019). To meet the needs of the child, PMIs can be adapted as single-case designs for individual support (Hanline et al., 2022) or in group settings for children with and without disabilities as to avoid "singling out" any children or removing them from settings (Hollingsworth, 2005).

In addition to positively impacting the presence, mastery, and confidence with prosocial skills (e.g., following rules, sharing, listening, taking turns, cooperating; Harjusola-Webb et al., 2012), PMIs have also been shown to have positive effects on decreasing classroom victimization and rejection against children experiencing neurodiversity or a medical condition (Devine et al., 2016). Children who have participated in PMIs have experienced improvements in increased levels of engagement as well as more social connections and larger friendship networks (Hanline et al., 2022; Harjusola-Webb et al., 2012), which also is associated with higher levels of peer acceptance and feelings of connectedness to school and classroom (Chang & Locke, 2016). With an increase in participation, communication, and connection alongside peers, it may be that PMIs can broadly decrease the impact of isolation and stigmatization among children with medical conditions and neurodiversity, improving aspects of their wellbeing.

Clinical, Policy, and Practical Applications and Implications

Findings discussed in this chapter have many implications for clinical practice and policy development. Given that early intervention can play a critical role in the development of peer relationships and interactions (Barbarin & Wasik, 2011), early childhood educational settings (e.g., preschool) may be one of most effective contexts for interventions to improve inclusion of children with youth with medical conditions and neurodivergent youth. Integrated classrooms may promote and foster development of prosocial behaviors for youth with medical conditions or neurodivergence. Further, typically developing children in these settings can model social skills and learn from building meaningful relationships with peers that have a medical condition/neurodivergent youth (Hanline et al., 2022). Early intervention to promote and foster inclusion may promote long-term social and emotional development, which can begin a positive social trajectory that continues to later years.

Since research has shown that peer relationships are often facilitated by the child's family (Lamb & Bornstein, 2013), it may be important for caregivers to play a central role in promoting inclusion of youth with medical conditions and neurodivergent youth within peer relationships and interactions. Caregivers may also provide education to their children regarding inclusion and development of peer relationships with youth with medical conditions or neurodivergence. Additionally, development of interventions that include caregivers and siblings of children with medical conditions or neurodivergence as facilitators helping to support social bids, group entry skills, and fostering a sense of efficacy about interpersonal skills may boost self-efficacy for peer interaction in youth with medical conditions and neurodivergent youth. Caregivers and siblings can model appropriate prosocial behaviors as well as appropriate non-verbal reactions, gestures, and responses. Caregivers could also connect with local hospitals or disability advocacy groups to find local opportunities to participate in adaptive sports, providing children with medical conditions the opportunity to develop peer relationships in that setting. Medical staff should check in with families to understand what activities their patients are (or are not) participating in and educate caregivers on misconceptions around avoiding participation due to health reasons, if appropriate. Youth with medical conditions or neurodivergence who are joining new social activities may benefit from PMIs to improve opportunities to interact with peers and gain confidence to approach and interact with others. Health professionals should continue to screen for friendship difficulties and isolation among youth with medical conditions and neurodivergent youth so that they can offer suggestions to facilitate peer support (such as joining clubs or extracurricular activities). Medical professionals could help facilitate interventions by contacting school staff in cases where children report a lack of connection to peers.

Current research on social support in youth with medical conditions and neurodivergent youth has important implications for future directions in policy and practice. One important consideration is the integration of interventions within educational systems. Much of a child's social development occurs within educational settings, as early as preschool (Gifford-Smith & Brownell, 2003; Parker et al., 2015); therefore, it could be beneficial for these interventions targeting peer relationships and interactions for youth with medical conditions/neurodivergent youth to be integrated into educational settings. Some research has identified that interventions targeting social skills development (e.g., prosocial behaviors) can be integrated into educational settings during structured times (e.g., recess, playtime), and can be brief (e.g., lasting 10–15 min; Gunning et al., 2019). Future policies may need to be developed and implemented to integrate effective interventions into classroom settings for youth with medical conditions and neurodivergent youth.

Limitations of Current Knowledge and Directions for Future Research

In view of the findings reviewed in this chapter, future research efforts are needed in several areas related to peer relationships and interactions among both youth with medical conditions and neurodivergent youth. Overall, there is a considerable paucity of research in the area of peer support for these children. Much of the existing research focuses solely on adolescents. This general research focus makes sense because, developmentally, adolescence is a period where youth increasingly depend on peers for support rather than family members. However, findings from research done with adolescents are difficult to generalize to young children. Social skills and interactions with peers for a child in preschool are very different from a child who is elementary aged or in high school. Existing studies do not stratify their samples by age which makes it difficult to generate conclusions about which interventions work best for certain age ranges. Future research should more intentionally design studies focused on younger children or stratify analyses by age to better capture the impact of peer support and interventions to promote social inclusion of children at different ages or developmental stages. Conducting research that considers children's developmental stages will increase the specificity of interventions, so they better fit children's needs and ability levels.

Most research examining interventions that promote peer relationships and interactions have shown that PMI are most effective for neurodivergent children diagnosed with developmental or intellectual disabilities (e.g., ASD, developmental delay, down syndrome; (Hanline et al., 2022; Reichow & Song, 2024). Much of the work on neurodivergent children has focused on ASD specifically. Some research with children with medical conditions has found effectiveness of PMIs for child brain tumor survivors and children with Type I Diabetes (Devine et al., 2016; Kazemi et al., 2016). In general, however, there is a need for social skills interventions and peer support interventions for children with other types of medical conditions and neurodivergent children with conditions other than ASD. Extending research to examine PMIs in different medical condition populations can provide pertinent information regarding how to best include children with medical conditions in peer relationships and interactions.

There is a large body of research that examines how peer support for medical-related issues (e.g., adherence, medical management) is beneficial for adolescents with medical conditions. However, this has not been extended to young children, and there is no research to our knowledge that examines how peers can support medical-specific sequelae for young children. Furthermore, results about the impact of social skills training on social competence are less clear for children with medical conditions. Some researchers argue that due to increased social isolation, children with medical conditions at this age fail to develop social skills comparable to healthy peers (Darcy et al., 2014, 2019; Fraser, 2003; McLoone et al., 2013; Tse et al., 2007; Willard et al., 2021). On the other hand, other researchers found no difference in social competence between children with medical conditions and healthy children and between children with different medical conditions (Nassau & Drotar, 1995; Noll et al., 2010). The unclear results may be due to the varied medical conditions experienced by children across studies. It also may be that, in some instances, children are learning social skills through interactions with the family rather than peers, particularly through interactions with parents and siblings. Thus, even if a child with a medical condition lacks opportunities for social experiences outside of the home, they can still develop social skills with members of the family unit, and this may account for equivocal findings in the research. Additionally, parents of children with medical conditions may realize the isolation their children face and are vigilant in ensuring opportunities for peer interaction to overcome absences from school and activities related to medical appointments and/or hospitalizations.

Our review of the literature indicated there has been limited consideration of the impact of condition severity on peer support and peer interaction for young children. Condition severity has not typically been considered when evaluating social skills and peer relationships in young children with medical conditions or neurodivergence. It has been shown that neurodivergent youth with more severe or profound disabilities engage less in peer interactions (Kuutti et al., 2022). Often, studies included children with particular conditions with mild impairments in the same sample as children with the same disorder with severe impairments (Nassau & Drotar, 1995). The level of impairment across different medical conditions and neurodevelopmental disabilities may be more predictive of similar challenges and experiences compared to within the same condition.

Many interventions cited utilized a single−case design, which limits generalizability (Chang & Locke, 2016; Gunning et al., 2019; Hanline et al., 2022). More rigorous designs with a larger study population are more likely to be disseminated widely and impact change. Study designs evaluating interventions for children with youth with medical conditions or neurodivergent youth should also try to include a comparison group of healthy or typically developing children. Across the board, research examining the effectiveness of interventions that promote social development among ethnically and culturally diverse samples is scarce. Most studies cited in this chapter have almost entirely white samples. Research efforts should be made to examine the challenges that this population may experience and the effectiveness of interventions for this population in ethnically and culturally diverse samples.

Conclusion

In this chapter we reviewed the importance of peer connection and support for young children with a particular focus on friendships and peer relationships among neurodivergent children or children with medical conditions. Research demonstrates the importance of peer relationships for children with these conditions because peer support can improve wellbeing and reduce negative symptoms, even among young children. Social skills development is an area for further study and intervention because it is the foundation for friendships as children age. PMIs designed to build social skills, particularly for neurodivergent children, hold promise but need to be tested more rigorously. We suggest that further consideration be given to integrating PMIs for young children into educational settings. We hope that this chapter serves as a call to action for further research targeting children with health conditions' peer engagement in both an exploratory and goal-oriented context.

References

af Sandeberg, M., Johansson, E., Björk, O., & Wettergren, L. (2008). Health-related quality of life relates to school attendance in children on treatment for cancer. *Journal of Pediatric Oncology Nursing, 25*(5), 265–274. https://doi.org/10.1177/1043454208321119

Baginsky, M. (2004). Peer support: Expectations and realities. *Pastoral Care in Education, 22*(1), 3–9. https://doi.org/10.1111/j.0264-3944.2004.00280.x

Barbarin, O., & Wasik, B. (2011). *Handbook of child development and early education: Research to practice*. Guilford Publications.

Barker, D., & Quittner, A. (2016). A biopsychosocial model of cystic fibrosis: Social and emotional functioning, adherence, and quality of life. In *Cystic fibrosis* (pp. 468–481). CRC Press.

Baron-Cohen, S., Leslie, A. M., & Frith, U. (1985). Does the autistic child have a "theory of mind" ? *Cognition, 21*(1), 37–46. https://doi.org/10.1016/0010-0277(85)90022-8

Brown, R. T. (2004). *Handbook of pediatric psychology in school settings*. Lawrence Erlbaum Associates.

Carter, R., Halawah, A., & Trinh, S. L. (2018). Peer exclusion during the pubertal transition: The role of social competence. *Journal of Youth and Adolescence, 47*(1), 121–134. https://doi.org/10.1007/s10964-017-0682-8

Chang, Y.-C., & Locke, J. (2016). A systematic review of peer-mediated interventions for children with autism spectrum disorder. *Research in Autism Spectrum Disorders, 27*, 1–10. https://doi.org/10.1016/j.rasd.2016.03.010

Christiansen, H. L., Bingen, K., Hoag, J. A., Karst, J. S., Velázquez-Martin, B., & Barakat, L. P. (2015). Providing children and adolescents opportunities for social interaction as a standard of care in pediatric oncology. *Pediatric Blood & Cancer, 62*(S5). https://doi.org/10.1002/pbc.25774

Chu, P. S., Saucier, D. A., & Hafner, E. (2010). Meta-analysis of the relationships between social support and wellbeing in children and adolescents. *Journal of Social and Clinical Psychology, 29*(6), 624–645. https://doi.org/10.1521/jscp.2010.29.6.624

Coleman, N., Sykes, W., & Groom, C. (2017). Peer support and children and young people's mental health: Research review. United Kingdom Department for Education. https://assets.publishing.service.gov.uk/media/5a820b3d40f0b62305b922c5/Children_and_young_people_s_mental_health_peer_support.pdf

Darcy, L., Björk, M., Enskär, K., & Knutsson, S. (2014). The process of striving for an ordinary, everyday life, in young children living with cancer, at six months and one year post diagnosis. *European Journal of Oncology Nursing, 18*(6), 605–612. https://doi.org/10.1016/j.ejon.2014.06.006

Darcy, L., Enskär, K., & Björk, M. (2019). Young children's experiences of living an everyday life with cancer—A three year interview study. *European Journal of Oncology Nursing, 39*, 1–9. https://doi.org/10.1016/j.ejon.2018.12.007

Devine, K. A., Bukowski, W. M., Sahler, O. J. Z., Ohman-Strickland, P., Smith, T. H., Lown, E. A., Patenaude, A. F., Korones, D. N., & Noll, R. B. (2016). Social competence in childhood brain tumor survivors: Feasibility and preliminary outcomes of a peer-mediated intervention. *Journal of Developmental & Behavioral Pediatrics, 37*(6), 475–482. https://doi.org/10.1097/DBP.0000000000000315

Ford, T. G., Kwon, K.-A., & Tsotsoros, J. D. (2021). Early childhood distance learning in the U.S. during the COVID pandemic: Challenges and opportunities. *Children and Youth Services Review, 131*, 106297. https://doi.org/10.1016/j.childyouth.2021.106297

Fraser, D. F. G. (2003). Strangers in their own land: Friendship issues when children have cancer. *Journal of Research in Special Educational Needs, 3*(3), 147–153. https://doi.org/10.1111/1471-3802.00009

Gifford-Smith, M. E., & Brownell, C. A. (2003). Childhood peer relationships: Social acceptance, friendships, and peer networks. *Journal of School Psychology, 41*(4), 235–284. https://doi.org/10.1016/S0022-4405(03)00048-7

Graham, L. J. (2023). *Inclusive education for the 21st century: Theory, policy and practice* (2nd ed.). Routledge. https://doi.org/10.4324/9781003350897

Gunning, C., Breathnach, Ó., Holloway, J., McTiernan, A., & Malone, B. (2019). A systematic review of peer-mediated interventions for preschool children with autism Spectrum disorder in inclusive settings. *Review Journal of Autism and Developmental Disorders, 6*(1), 40–62. https://doi.org/10.1007/s40489-018-0153-5

Hanline, M. F., Eldridge, J. N., & Robbins, A. (2022). Including peers in intervention for young children with disabilities: A systematic review of single case design studies. *Infants & Young Children, 35*(3), 165–188. https://doi.org/10.1097/IYC.0000000000000221

Harjusola-Webb, S., Hubbell, S. P., & Bedesem, P. (2012). Increasing prosocial behaviors of young children with disabilities in inclusive classrooms using a combination of peer-mediated intervention and social narratives. *Beyond Behavior, 21*(2), 29–36.

Hollingsworth, H. L. (2005). Interventions to promote peer social interactions in preschool settings. *Young Exceptional Children, 9*(1), 2–11. https://doi.org/10.1177/109625060500900101

Hoyne, C., & Egan, S. M. (2024). Exploring the role of home play and learning activities in socioemotional development at 36-months: Findings from a large birth cohort study. *Infant Behavior and Development*, *77*, 1–24. https://doi.org/10.1016/j.infbeh.2024.102000

Johnson, E., Atkinson, P., Muggeridge, A., Cross, J. H., & Reilly, C. (2021). Inclusion and participation of children with epilepsy in schools: Views of young people, school staff and parents. *Seizure, 93*, 34–43. https://doi.org/10.1016/j.seizure.2021.10.007

Kazemi, S., Parvizy, S., Atlasi, R., & Baradaran, H. R. (2016). Evaluating the effectiveness of peer-based intervention in managing type I diabetes mellitus among children and adolescents: A systematic review. *Medical Journal of the Islamic Republic of Iran, 30*, 442.

Koller, D., Pouesard, M. L., & Rummens, J. A. (2018). Defining social inclusion for children with disabilities: A critical literature review. *Children & Society, 32*(1), 1–13. https://doi.org/10.1111/chso.12223

Kuutti, T., Sajaniemi, N., Björn, P. M., Heiskanen, N., & Reunamo, J. (2022). Participation, involvement and peer relationships in children with special educational needs in early childhood education. *European Journal of Special Needs Education, 37*(4), 587–602. https://doi.org/10.1080/08856257.2021.1920214

La Greca, A. M., & Harrison, H. M. (2005). Adolescent peer relations, friendships, and romantic relationships: Do they predict social anxiety and depression? *Journal of Clinical Child & Adolescent Psychology, 34*(1), 49–61. https://doi.org/10.1207/s15374424jccp3401_5

La Greca, A. M., Bearman, K. J., & Moore, H. (2002). Peer relations of youth with pediatric conditions and health risks: Promoting social support and healthy lifestyles. *Journal of Developmental & Behavioral Pediatrics, 23*(4), 271.

Lamb, M. E., & Bornstein, M. H. (2013). *Social and personality development: An advanced textbook*. Taylor and Francis.

Malik, F., & Marwaha, R. (2022). Developmental stages of social emotional development in children. In *StatPearls*. StatPearls Publishing. https://www.ncbi.nlm.nih.gov/books/NBK534819/

Martinez, W., Carter, J. S., & Legato, L. J. (2011). Social competence in children with chronic illness: A meta-analytic review. *Journal of Pediatric Psychology, 36*(8), 878–890. https://doi.org/10.1093/jpepsy/jsr035

Martiniuk, A., Silva, M., Amylon, M., & Barr, R. (2014). Camp programs for children with cancer and their families: Review of research progress over the past decade. *Pediatric Blood & Cancer, 61*(5), 778–787. https://doi.org/10.1002/pbc.24912

McLoone, J. K., Wakefield, C. E., & Cohn, R. J. (2013). Childhood cancer survivors' school (re)entry: Australian parents' perceptions: School (re)entry after childhood cancer. *European Journal of Cancer Care, 22*(4), 484–492. https://doi.org/10.1111/ecc.12054

Nassau, J. H., & Drotar, D. (1995). Social competence in children with IDDM and asthma: Child, teacher, and parent reports of children's social adjustment, social performance, and social skills. *Journal of Pediatric Psychology, 20*(2), 187–204. https://doi.org/10.1093/jpepsy/20.2.187

National Association for the Education of & Young Children & Division for Early Childhood. (2009). *Early childhood inclusion.* http://www.dec-sped.org/uploads/docs/about_dec/position_concept_papers/PositionStatement_Inclusion_Joint_updated_May2009.pdf

Nijs, S., Vlaskamp, C., & Maes, B. (2016). The nature of peer-directed behaviours in children with profound intellectual and multiple disabilities and its relationship with social scaffolding behaviours of the direct support worker. *Child: Care, Health and Development, 42*(1), 98–108. https://doi.org/10.1111/cch.12295

Noll, R. B., Kiska, R., Reiter-Purtill, J., Gerhardt, C. A., & Vannatta, K. (2010). A controlled, longitudinal study of the social functioning of youth with sickle cell disease. *Pediatrics, 125*(6), e1453–e1459. https://doi.org/10.1542/peds.2009-2996

Odar, C., Canter, K. S., & Roberts, M. C. (2013). Relationship between camp attendance and self-perceptions in children with chronic health conditions: A meta-analysis. *Journal of Pediatric Psychology, 38*(4), 398–411. https://doi.org/10.1093/jpepsy/jss176

Odom, S. L., & Strain, P. S. (1984). Peer-mediated approaches to promoting children's social interaction: A review. *American Journal of Orthopsychiatry, 54*(4), 544–557. https://doi.org/10.1111/j.1939-0025.1984.tb01525.x

Parker, J. G., Rubin, K. H., Erath, S. A., Wojslawowicz, J. C., & Buskirk, A. A. (2015). Peer relationships, child development, and adjustment: A developmental psychopathology perspective. In D. Cicchetti & D. J. Cohen (Eds.), *Developmental psychopathology* (1st ed., pp. 419–493). Wiley. https://doi.org/10.1002/9780470939383.ch12

Pawlowski, C., Buckman, C., Tumin, D., Smith, A. W., & Crotty, J. (2019). National Trends in pediatric headache and associated functional limitations. *Clinical Pediatrics, 58*(14), 1502–1508. https://doi.org/10.1177/0009922819875560

Petry, K., & Maes, B. (2007). Description of the support needs of people with profound multiple disabilities using the 2002 AAMR system: An overview of literature. *Education and Training in Developmental Disabilities, 42*(2), 130–143.

Plage, S., Kuskoff, E., Hoang, N.-P., & Povey, J. (2022). Educational participation of primary school children with cancer from a Life Course perspective: A critical review of the literature. *International Journal of Educational Research, 114*, 101990. https://doi.org/10.1016/j.ijer.2022.101990

Reichow, B., & Song, J. (2024). Overview of reviews of peer-mediated interventions for young children with disabilities. *Topics in Early Childhood Special Education*, 02711214241281383. https://doi.org/10.1177/02711214241281383.

Rubin, K. H., & Ross, H. S. (2012). *Peer relationships and social skills in childhood*. Springer Science & Business Media.

Shalaby, R. A. H., & Agyapong, V. I. O. (2020). Peer support in mental health: Literature review. *JMIR Mental Health, 7*(6), e15572. https://doi.org/10.2196/15572

Stewart, D., & Sun, J. (2004). How can we build resilience in primary school aged children? The importance of social support from adults and peers in family, school and community settings. *Asia Pacific Journal of Public Health, 16*(1_suppl), 37–41. https://doi.org/10.1177/101053950401600S10

Thirumanickam, A., Raghavendra, P., & Olsson, C. (2011). Participation and social networks of school-age children with complex communication needs: A descriptive study. *Augmentative and Alternative Communication, 27*(3), 195–204. https://doi.org/10.3109/07434618.2011.610818

Tse, E., Hamiwka, L., Sherman, E. M. S., & Wirrell, E. (2007). Social skills problems in children with epilepsy: Prevalence, nature and predictors. *Epilepsy & Behavior, 11*(4), 499–505. https://doi.org/10.1016/j.yebeh.2007.08.008

Uslu, F., & Gizir, S. (2017). School belonging of adolescents: The role of teacher–student relationships, peer relationships and family involvement. *Educational Sciences: Theory & Practice, 17*, 63–82. https://doi.org/10.12738/estp.2017.1.0104

Van Der Laan, S. E. I., Berkelbach Van Der Sprenkel, E. E., Lenters, V. C., Finkenauer, C., Van Der Ent, C. K., & Nijhof, S. L. (2023). Defining and measuring resilience in children with a chronic disease: A scoping review. *Adversity and Resilience Science, 4*(2), 105–123. https://doi.org/10.1007/s42844-023-00092-2

Van Der Meulen, K., Granizo, L., & Del Barrio, C. (2021). Emotional peer support interventions for students with SEND: A systematic review. *Frontiers in Psychology, 12*, 797913. https://doi.org/10.3389/fpsyg.2021.797913

Van Harmelen, A.-L., Gibson, J. L., St Clair, M. C., Owens, M., Brodbeck, J., Dunn, V., Lewis, G., Croudace, T., Jones, P. B., Kievit, R. A., & Goodyer, I. M. (2016). Friendships and family support reduce subsequent depressive symptoms in at-risk adolescents. *PLoS One, 11*(5), e0153715. https://doi.org/10.1371/journal.pone.0153715

Webster-Stratton, C., & Reid, M. J. (2004). Strengthening social and emotional competence in young children—The foundation for early school readiness and success: Incredible years classroom social skills and problem-solving curriculum. *Infants & Young Children, 17*(2), 96–113. https://doi.org/10.1097/00001163-200404000-00002

Willard, V. W., Gordon, M. L., Means, B., Brennan, R. C., Conklin, H. M., Merchant, T. E., Vinitsky, A., & Harman, J. L. (2021). Social emotional functioning in preschool-aged children with cancer: Comparisons between children with brain and non-CNS solid tumor. *Journal of Pediatric Psychology, 46*(7), 790–800. https://doi.org/10.1093/jpepsy/jsab018
Woodhead, M., Faulkner, D., Littleton, K., & Open University. (1999). *Making sense of social development*. Routledge in Association with the Open University.

Chapter 9
Fostering Resilience in Children with Chronic Illnesses During and After Hospitalization

Margaret E. Wazevich, Riley I. Justice, and Laura Nabors

Abstract This chapter discusses the complex challenges faced by children with chronic illnesses, many of whom have developmental disabilities, during and after hospitalization. Drawing on Bronfenbrenner's Ecological Systems Theory, it underscores the value of a holistic system-of-care approach. Hospitalization can disrupt daily routines, leading to social isolation, anxiety, and academic difficulties. Effective interventions include peer support and mentorship programs that foster resilience, belonging, and emotional well-being, along with family-to-family connections that offer guidance and validation. Psychoeducation and cognitive-behavioral therapies help families cope and improve functioning. School achievement is supported through hospital school programs, technology-assisted learning, and reintegration strategies that accommodate medical needs and build peer understanding. Collaboration among families, healthcare providers, and schools is crucial for medical regimen adherence, guided by tailored plans and ongoing communication. The chapter highlights gaps in research and calls for more studies on interventions that best promote resilience and quality of life for affected children.

Keywords Children with chronic illnesses · Emotional support · Parent support · EHealth · Hospital school programs · School reintegration programs · Teacher support · Adherence · Schooling during hospitalization

There has been an increase in the number of children who have chronic illnesses (Compas et al., 2012; Wijlaars et al., 2016). This is due to increasing prevalence of illnesses, increased survival rates, and the fact that health care professionals are becoming better at identifying and treating chronic illnesses (Forrest et al., 2025). Rates vary across studies; however, it is estimated that 10–20% of children have a chronic illness (Baker & Claridge, 2023; Kohl & Barnett, 2020). Some define

M. E. Wazevich · R. I. Justice · L. Nabors (✉)
School of Human Services, College of Education, Criminal Justice, Human Services, and Information Technology, University of Cincinnati, Cincinnati, OH, USA
e-mail: naborsla@ucmail.uc.edu

L. Nabors and T. Stanton-Chapman (eds.), *Developmental Disabilities and Chronic Illness in Young Children*, Springer Series on Child and Family Studies,
https://doi.org/10.1007/978-3-032-08523-8_9

chronic illnesses in broad terms—as involving physical, behavioral, developmental, or mental health conditions lasting more than 3 months and can require hospitalization (Baker & Claridge, 2023; Mokkink et al., 2008). It is important to understand psychosocial and school interventions and outcomes of treatment for this vulnerable group of children to improve their quality of life. Children with chronic health conditions whose educational progress is impacted by their illness are eligible for special education services (i.e.,: 504 Plan or Individualized Education Plan) under the category of Other Health Impairment (OHI). In this chapter, our focus is on children with chronic illnesses, such as asthma, cancer, congenital heart conditions, or diabetes, who often face hospitalization and have high use of healthcare services (Barrio-Cortes et al., 2024).

Children with chronic illnesses experience challenges that significantly impact their physical, emotional, social, and academic well-being (Baker & Claridge, 2023; Steinke et al., 2016). Chronic illnesses frequently disrupt normal routines which can lead to psychosocial challenges that extend beyond the medical condition (Douma et al., 2021; Rohan & Verma, 2020). These challenges include feelings of marginalization, social isolation, and uncertainty about the future (Lum et al., 2019). Our orientation is also one emphasizing context, as the child is embedded in the context of the family, medical care team, and school. Addressing children's needs requires psychoeducation, support from peers and the medical team, and school programs to enhance the child's overall quality of life (Merianos et al., 2015; Caggiano et al., 2021).

Theory and Rationale

Bronfenbrenner's Ecological Systems Theory (1977; Guy-Evans, 2024) states that an individual's development is a product of the interconnected environmental systems that surround them. Similarly, Rolland (1987) proposed that an individual's chronic illness interacts with the systems in which they are embedded. These systems include the parent-child unit, family, hospital, and school. A system of care is necessary to address the immediate and long-term impacts of chronic illness to provide holistic care that addresses the physical aspects of illness and the emotional and social dimensions. In this chapter, we review interventions to improve child and parent support and coping. We also discuss school support for these children. Educational support services and using technology to provide academic resources can improve academic performance. Moreover, flexibility in communication with the child and parent(s), and in teaching materials, can assist in ensuring learning as children cope with school absences and complications. Psychoeducational interventions, peer support groups, parent support, and support of academic progress are crucial for addressing challenges faced by children who cope with illness-related hospitalizations. These interventions support the child's emotional resilience and encourage the development and feelings of confidence in disease management, which are vital for managing health conditions independently (Caggiano et al., 2021; Merianos et al., 2015).

Peer Support

Peer support programs have been shown to be highly effective in helping children with chronic illness develop resilience by fostering a sense of connection, belonging, and sense of well-being (Merianos et al., 2016; Olsson et al., 2005). These programs often involve mentorship, typically pairing hospitalized children with older or more experienced patients who have gone through similar experiences (Wiemann et al., 2019). Mentors provide emotional support, share coping strategies that worked for them, and offer guidance on managing medical care, hospital experiences, and coping with a medical illness at school and in the community (Wiemann et al., 2019). Peer mentorship programs provide children with a valuable source of social support from others facing similar challenges and provide a source for medication information (Lewis et al., 2016; Merianos et al., 2016). Peer programs can create a sense of community allowing children to see that they are not alone in their struggles and that others have successfully navigated similar challenges. The bonds formed through peer mentorship programs can also persist beyond the hospital stay, continuing to offer emotional and social support as children face future challenges related to their illness (Kirk & Milnes, 2021). For example, Nationwide Children's Hospital has a family-to-family (F2F) program in which families with children with medical needs are provided the opportunity to speak with another parent/guardian or adult patient who has been through something similar. The peer mentor is meant to listen to the family's story, provide personal perspectives and wisdom, validate the family's concerns and feelings, and guide them through the hospital system as an experienced patient (Nationwide Children's, 2025). This family mentorship model has been used in various other hospitals such as the Children's Hospital of Philadelphia (Kratchman et al., 2015), Stollery Children's Hospital (Wodinski et al., 2017), and the Association for Children's Mental Health in Michigan (Anthony et al., 2019).

Diabetes is the second most common chronic illness among youth (Hill et al., 2019; Organized camping, an effective mentorship program, has become more specialized in regard to meeting the needs of youth with specific chronic illnesses. For example, there is evidence from research within diabetes camps that peer support is beneficial for younger children, and that they learn new information to manage their disease in supportive settings (Hill et al., 2019). Collaborating with a local university, a local hospital's center for diabetes, and the Lions Club, a family diabetes camp was created to guide children and adolescents in managing their condition. Parent(s)/guardian(s) reported a positive increase of perceptions of their child's resiliency, campers reported that they learned about crucial issues, such as independence and medication management, and addressed family concerns regarding motivation, community, and challenges of the health condition. Mixed methods studies and randomized controlled trials are needed to understand which features of support groups are most effective and determine the psychological impact of these groups (Kirk & Milnes, 2021).

Lewis et al. (2016) evaluated youth perceptions of a peer support program, based in Australia, for adolescents with a variety of chronic illnesses. The program served youth 12 years and older and involved attending social events and camps. Lewis et al. (2016) used focus groups and surveys to assess the impact of the program. Qualitative data from the focus groups indicated that ongoing membership was related to feelings of support from others facing similar challenges. However, analyses of survey responses did not show change in distress levels or self-esteem. This program was for older youth, and more research is needed to determine the effectiveness of support groups for younger children.

Supporting Parents

Support for parents is intertwined with family coping and support of the child. Parent support is critical for some parents, as they may experience anxiety and depression associated with supporting their child and family "through" their child's illness (Cohn et al., 2020). Lancaster et al. (2023) reviewed studies (between 2011 through 2020) of families with a child with a disability or chronic illness to examine whether support programs improved parent well-being (e.g., hope, gratitude, stress were assessed). The programs they reviewed had a support component and were delivered either online or in community settings. Families with children under 18 years were included in the studies. Programs that offered support groups (meeting weekly or at times less frequently) could reduce parental anxiety and depression, while concomitantly improving variables related to positive coping (e.g., hope; Lancaster et al., 2023). Results were not always clear-cut, however, and programs offered other interventions for parents and the family, making it difficult to tell if support from other parents was driving positive change or another intervention component was responsible for change. More research is needed to uncover how support impacts the parents and then is translated to positive support of the child, uplifting child emotional functioning.

Interventions to Promote Child Functioning

During a hospital stay, children often experience a wide range of emotions, from anxiety about medical procedures to sadness or frustration about being away from home. Emotional regulation techniques, such as deep breathing, progressive muscle relaxation, and guided imagery, can help children manage these emotions and reduce the psychological burden of their illness (Catanzano et al., 2020; Compas et al., 2012). Although not a primary emphasis of this chapter, the techniques are also helpful for coping with pain (Nabbijohn et al. 2021). Boyd and Hunsberger (1998) suggested several strategies, which work in the hospital and when the child returns home, such as: (1) allowing emotional expression, (2) explaining procedures (in developmentally appropriate terms), and (3) trying to provide the child some control over what is happening. They also recommended: using distraction, cognitive restructuring (to move to a more positive outlook) and a problem-solving approach. The family should receive education, as it promotes child resilience in that children can have confidence that they will receive good medical care at home. Child therapists and the medical team can also teach coping skills (for coping with procedures, pain, and stress). Compas et al. (2012) proposed that children who are taught specific coping strategies, such as problem-solving, emotional regulation, and mindfulness, are better able to manage the stress and anxiety associated with hospitalization.

Day et al. (2020) reviewed randomized controlled trials of 25 psychoeducational interventions, often delivered in groups or clinics. Interventions typically provided education about pathophysiology of the disease, triggers for symptoms, taking medications, coping with disease flare-ups, and improving healthy lifestyles. Day et al. (2020) mentioned that most interventions focused on youth with asthma and diabetes. Additionally, information on how to educate children in minority groups and children and families living in poverty will be important to move the field forward.

Sattoe et al. (2015) reviewed studies focusing on self-management of disease from 2003 to 2014, with youth ranging between seven through 25 years of age. A wide range of chronic illnesses were represented and 78 studies (primarily randomized controlled trials and cohort studies, with some qualitative studies) were presented. Many different interventions were used, including improving emotional and social skills, goal setting, problem–solving, and teaching skills for managing symptoms of illnesses. Typically, children and parents had parallel skill-building sessions. Education was provided to children in many ways—using technology, videos, comic books, role play, goal-setting activities, art, peer to peer education, and homework assignments. Table 9.1 presents some of the interventions used in studies reviewed by Sattoe et al. (2015), and it is noteworthy that these strategies are reflected in other studies (e.g., Catanzano et al., 2020; Compas et al., 2012; Nabbijohn et al. 2021).

Table 9.1 Interventions included in studies focusing on disease management

Area	Skills
Social skills	Social initiation, coping with teasing and bullying, explaining condition to others, coping in relationships with peers
Emotional skills	Increasing self-esteem, sharing feelings, increasing positive thoughts, stress management
Goal setting	Action plans, goal development, motivational interviewing
Communication	Family discussion, problem-solving, sharing ideas with family
Disease management	Adherence to the regimen, understanding the disease [symptoms, triggers for flare-ups of symptoms; disease course], review of steps for disease management

EHealth

Interventions may be delivered online, and this may be a great way to connect for children and families who do not have time to attend interventions offered at hospitals or other outpatient clinics or offices. Thabrew et al. (2018) reviewed randomized controlled trials of Ehealth interventions from 1997 to 2017 for children ages 10–18 with a variety of chronic illnesses to determine the impact of these interventions on child anxiety, depression, and quality of life. Ehealth interventions were related to reductions in anxiety and depression, which is positive. Results on change in quality of life were equivocal, indicating a need for further study of Ehealth interventions to determine if they are related to improved perceptions of quality of life or well-being. In part, it may have been difficult to understand effectiveness because of the many interventions that are offered (e.g., behavioral therapies, CBT, mindfulness and other cognitive therapies, acceptance and commitment therapy; Thabrew et al., 2018). Given all the child, family, illness-related, and therapy-related factors, research is needed to understand which components of online therapies work for whom and how they work, so these interventions can be replicated.

Interventions to Promote Parent Functioning

Law et al. (2019) reviewed 44 randomized controlled trials of interventions presenting psychological therapies for parents of children who had chronic illnesses (diabetes, asthma, traumatic brain injury, cancer and chronic pain were conditions of interest). They found that both cognitive-behavioral therapies (CBT) and problem-solving (PS) therapies assisted parents and had potential to improve child behavioral issues (e.g., maladaptive behaviors), whereas results of motivational interviewing (using encouragement and goal setting) and family therapies were less clear-cut. Law et al. (2019) defined these therapies as follows:

> CBT - … treatment is focused on altering maladaptive social/environmental, behavioral, and cognitive factors in order to reduce symptoms (chiefly of child behavioral problems) and prevent relapse. (Law et al., 2019, p. 9)
>
> PS - … emphasizes the role of constructive problem-solving attitudes and skills in fostering enhanced social competence and reduced emotional distress. Steps include: defining the problem, generating alternative solutions, decision making, and solution implementation and evaluation. (Law et al., 2019, p. 9)

Results were not conclusive in studies for children with asthma, and results varied based on type of therapy for the other chronic illnesses. However, in general, CBT had a positive impact on child behaviors, while not always impacting child mental health or family outcomes. In contrast, PS did not strongly impact child outcomes (i.e., child behaviors and mental health). Nonetheless, PS did help parents with parenting and had a small positive influence on parental mental health. The researchers conducting the review did note that more information is needed to determine if change is maintained over the long-term (Law et al., 2019). Other therapies, such as motivational interviewing and family therapies need more investigation to determine if they have a positive impact on child behavior and mental health as well as on parent behavior mental health. Koumarianou et al. (2021) reviewed psychosocial interventions for children with cancer and found that CBT and PS interventions for families supported the child and family unit, providing further support for use of these interventions to improve care of children and families.

Results of another meta-analysis, conducted by Doupnik et al. (2017) revealed support for interventions to improve parent functioning while a child is hospitalized. Doupnik et al. (2017) reviewed 32 studies (16 of which were with parents in the neonatal intensive care unit [NICU]). They included randomized controlled trials, quasi-experimental studies, and single group designs in their analysis. Interventions varied, addressing education to improve care of the child's illness, emotional self-care (e.g., encouraging adaptive emotional expression and self-care), and social support (i.e., support from others, such as nurses). Many interventions were multi-faceted, and social support was typically part of multi-component interventions. Most interventions were delivered while parents were in the hospital, although a few began before hospitalization of the child. Interventions in emergency room situations (e.g., NICU) typically had emotional self-care components for parents. Interventions, especially those involving emotional self-care, were related to reductions in parental anxiety, depression, and stress, but in some studies results were equivocal. Child outcomes were assessed in one-third of the studies, and results indicated reductions in negative child behaviors if parents participated in supportive interventions. About a third of the studies examined family outcomes and parent interventions could result in improved parent-child interactions and improved family functioning. Doupnik et al. (2017) cautioned that despite positive results, it was difficult to obtain reimbursement for parent support interventions, and researchers need to continue to assess child outcomes to provide evidence of the value of these interventions.

When providing supportive interventions for parents and the family unit, healthcare professionals need to assess child, parent, and family functioning (using interviews, observations, surveys) to determine if family therapy, with a trained mental health professional, is warranted to address how the dynamics of the child's chronic illness interact with family patterns and coping (Sansom-Daly et al., 2012). Assigning a social worker or psychologist to work with families is one way to assess individual family needs for support. Engaging in family therapy may be a more intensive endeavor, individualized to family needs, that in the long-term will improve family interaction patterns, dynamics, and communication, leading to improved family functioning.

Educational Support

Hospitalization can amplify the difficulties faced by children with chronic illnesses. Children with chronic health conditions often have difficulty attending school regularly due to hospitalizations or medical treatments (Barnett et al., 2020; Wikel & Markelz, 2023). Extended hospital stays interrupt academic progress and social connections and create feelings of loss regarding independence and normalcy (Hu et al., 2022). Integrated psychological and academic services in pediatric hospital settings, which combine educational support and psychological care to holistically address the academic, emotional, and medical needs of children with complex chronic conditions have been shown to be effective (Marshall et al., 2022). In the next sections of this chapter, we review interventions to promote school functioning.

Technology-Assisted Learning

Technology-assisted learning enables children with chronic illness to continue their education remotely through meetings with teachers (on Zoom) and learning through educational videos and games. Also, there are websites with tutorials and educational materials that can support parents in tutoring their children, if teachers are difficult to reach with questions. Technology-assisted learning, using apps or games for example, is a critical tool for students with chronic medical conditions, enabling them to maintain academic progress and stay connected to their school community during hospitalizations or recovery at home through flexible, personalized, and remote learning options (Edwards et al., 2021). Additionally, multi-modal digital game-based learning has been helpful for children with chronic illnesses in increasing social interaction and academic motivation (Chin & Tsuei, 2014).

Hospital School Programs

Hospital schools provide a unique opportunity for students to continue their education while simultaneously receiving medical treatment. Teachers can provide individualized lessons in the hospital setting (Caggiano, 2021). Other hospitals can have "schools" (classrooms at the hospital) where teachers have office hours and are able to teach small groups of children. Hospital schools can prevent disengagement from school, education, and learning (Barnett et al., 2020). Moreover, hospital school programs provide continuity in education during hospitalization, aiming to ensure hospitalized students have equal opportunities as their peers until they can return to school. These programs maintain academic engagement, prevent negative consequences of school absenteeism, and ensure that students can keep up with their peers academically (Caggiano et al., 2021). Moreover, a recent study found that being engaged in school while hospitalized improved child mood and children showed decreases pain and physiological distress after participating in lessons (Ciucci et al., 2024).

In addition to academic support, hospital school programs also provide emotional and psychological support to children during their hospital stay (Di Padova et al., 2024; Shaw & McCabe, 2008). For many children, being hospitalized can be a frightening and isolating experience. The hospital school environment increases a sense of connection to the outside world and community. By maintaining schoolwork and social interactions in the hospital, children experience less disruption to their routines, which promotes their mental well-being and emotional resilience. The academic and social engagement provided by hospital school programs is essential for maintaining the child's sense of identity as a student and reduces the psychological impact of being in the hospital (Emerson et al., 2016).

Reintegration Programs

School reintegration programs (e.g., programs that support children returning to school, with consultation from medical teams) can help reduce feelings of concern over the revolving door that can occur should a child require multiple hospitalizations, requiring multiple instances of school re-entry (Leite et al., 2023). Hospital–to–school reintegration programs focus on engaging children in school (e.g., developing plans for completing missed work and engaging in school during the recovery period after hospitalization) and promoting academic performance (Caggiano et al., 2021; Carlton et al., 2021). Consultation with the medical team can enhance abilities to follow the medical regimen at school and develop accommodations to help the child (e.g., taking the elevator and not the stairs if the child needs time to improve his/her stamina). These programs enhance academic achievement and decrease levels of depression among children who are returning to school (Helms et al., 2016). Another helpful feature of these programs can be improving understanding of the illness for peers in the classroom, affording them knowledge and advice for ways to engage with a child with a chronic illness (Canter & Roberts, 2012).

A multidisciplinary approach that includes educators, parent(s)/guardian(s), and healthcare professionals can ensure that children can return to school with less anxiety, more confidence, and a better understanding of their illness, which will improve their academic outcomes (Harden et al., 2020). Involving parents in the transition process is crucial to ensuring the child's emotional needs are met and ensures there is continuity of care. It is recommended that schools designate an individual to function as coordinator of student records (i.e.,: academic records, special education documents, etc.; Harden et al., 2020). When school nurses serve as liaisons with the child's medical team, they can infuse health care knowledge in educational plans and result in successful re–integration into the school (McCabe et al., 2021). We recommend a patient- and family-centered framework, to guide planning and implementation of comprehensive interventions for youth during re-integration. Including mental health, nursing, social work, and the child's medical team in planning can assist in designing plans to facilitate child social-emotional functioning, educational, and recreational needs.

Special Education Planning

Students with chronic health conditions may have needs for accommodations or modifications to their academic work, often necessitating the implementation of a Section 504 Plan or an Individualized Education Plan (IEP; Matthews, 2024). An IEP is a written document in which teachers, parents, school administrators, related services personnel, and students (when appropriate) collaborate to design a tailored educational program for a student with a disability. The Individuals with Disabilities Education Improvement Act of 2004 (IDEA) guides the delivery of special education supports and services for students (U.S. Department of Education, 2006). Typically, students with chronic illnesses who qualify for an IEP often fall under the category of Other Health Impairment, (OHI; NASET, 2008). Section 504 provides a broad spectrum of protections against discrimination because of disability, protecting the child's right to general or special education aids and services for their educational needs. A 504 plan also requires that students with disabilities have equal opportunities and access to athletics and extracurricular activities (Matthews, 2024). The major difference between a 504 plan and an IEP is that a 504 plan is meant for students with disabilities or chronic health conditions who do not require special education services (due to academic performance), whereas a student with an IEP (where a student's educational performance is below average levels) is most often in a special education classroom or program (Kassab & Claybourn, 2023; Schultz, 2020).

Harden et al. (2020) recommend teachers, parents, counselors, school health teams, and hospital teams collaborate to consider the impact of chronic symptoms and treatment on academic performance. Having an IEP (typically for being other health impaired) or 504 plan is developed when a child is falling behind academically (shows decrease in performance) and allows for easier academic adaptations and updates for the student's evolving medical situation and ensures teachers have the most up-to-date information regarding the student's health condition (Harden et al., 2020). Parents often become experts on their children to ensure their well-being (Baker & Claridge, 2023). This expertise can be extended to ensure that child illnesses are supported through special education plans (Individual Education Plans or Section 504 plans; Spiel et al., 2014) in schools or through homeschooling, as parent(s) may be more comfortable managing the child's illness at home.

Teachers have reported that when they had students with chronic illnesses, they were able to prepare better when the student had an IEP or a 504 plan (Matthews, 2024). Having a history of accommodations on record assisted educators in understanding what strategies had been used in the past to support the student (Matthews,

2024). If the medical team can consult during an IEP or 504 meeting, interventions can be developed, modified, or improved based on their input. At times, their feedback is instrumental in gaining additional services such as psychotherapy, physical therapy, or occupational therapy (Harden et al., 2020).

Adherence to the Medical Regimen

When considering the impact of interventions for children and their families, health professionals must think about adherence to the medical regimen (Kvarnström et al., 2021; Rohan & Verma, 2020). School professionals and therapists need to stay in contact with and be informed by the medical team, and this includes the child and parents as team members, to ensure that interventions are designed to facilitate adherence to taking medications or to following other aspects of the medical regimen (e.g., referrals for additional therapies). For many children ensuring medications are dispensed is enough, but others may need other therapies (e.g., psychotherapy, occupational therapy) or need to have other accommodations, such as modifying participation in physical education classes, having two sets of books (one for school and the other to use at home, because it is difficult to carry books home) or using elevators to get to classes on different floors in the school building. Involving the school nurse as a liaison to the medical team or involving a school-based therapist or school psychologist as a liaison may improve communication with the medical team (Kvarnström et al., 2021). Moreover, when medical providers establish trust in their relationship with the child and family, they improve their foundation from which to address adherence issues, and regular communication and support of the child and family can increase this trust.

We recommend a fivefold process to ensure a client- and family-focused approach to "planning for" adherence: (1) consult with the medical providers about medication and medical regimen, (2) consult with child and family—check feelings about and abilities to adhere to the regimen in different settings, (3) develop a plan—steps to facilitate adherence in the setting (home, school, sports, extracurriculars), (4) write down the plan, and (5) have checkpoints to ensure the plan is followed or updated as needed. Because the planning and monitoring of adherence is inextricably tied to family functioning, health professionals need to assess family abilities to understand and adhere to the medical regimen and make referrals for support—from support groups, medical professionals, and therapists (Psihogios et al., 2019; Rohan & Verma, 2020).

Case Study: Interviews to Assess Parent and Child Perceptions of Schooling During Hospitalizations

Our work is based on how the child with a chronic illness and parents cope with schooling as the illness takes a "center role" in the child and family journey—during hospitalizations which interrupt day-to-day routines and functioning. Parents mentioned that assisting their child with work on school assignments, helped their child to move forward with schoolwork and promoted feelings of achievement while in the hospital. In this case study, we review findings from our research (Wazevich et al., 2024). Children with chronic illnesses, siblings, and caregivers (most often parents, so parents will be used in this section of our chapter) participated in semi-structured interviews where they discussed how children were doing with school during a hospital stay for the child who had chronic illness. The children had a range of illnesses from cancer to medical issues associated with neurodevelopmental disabilities. Interviews were collected during activity groups (usually 60–75 min) at a local Ronald McDonald House (RMH), and children participated in art activities during their interviews. Approximately 30 parents and about 15 children with chronic illnesses and siblings participated in the interviews. Our project focused primarily on children aged 13 and younger, and therefore, the findings might not apply to the academic concerns of older children. Coders used an open-coding approach with several coders (to allow for triangulation of findings), and identified several themes such as child needs for homeschooling, missing friends, difficulties with school re-entry after hospitalization, and the importance of teacher support and availability to keep up with work. Information related to our interviews is discussed in the following paragraphs (Wazevich et al., 2024).

Children were keeping up with schoolwork, although some needed individual education planning to support their academic and medical needs and others were enrolled in homeschooling, because parents were unsure as to whether the school could meet the medical management needs for their child. Most parents reported that their child was on track academically and completing assignments. Part of this was due to flexibility of teachers, who provided "just the necessary" work and did not send "busy work." Thus, children were doing the critical assignments and getting the learning they needed to advance, and teachers were available via email, cellular telephone, or text messaging if there were questions. Teachers were there to help and support children, and a hallmark feature of the interviews was that teachers were making things work for the child. Flexibility on the part of teachers, in terms of texting and emailing parents when needed to provide incidental teaching opportunities (to teach information when needed) was highly valued by parents. They often served as tutors and advisors, helping children with their work. Children and parents reported appreciating a "lightened" workload, where children focused on the basics of "catching up" on critical academic material. Children and parents were tired, and children had limited resources, and therefore, focusing on the basics—what was needed to keep up with the class and learn—facilitated learning.

Several of the parents reported that returning to school after being at the RMH could be difficult. For example, one ten-year-old female, with an inflammatory bowel disease stated attending school after a hospitalization could be taxing because of "catching up" on missed classwork and having difficulty rotating between classes and finding books during the time when she was moving from class to class. A subset of children with chronic illnesses mentioned that they did not want to return to school, because they did not feel that other children understood their illness or because there were bullies in the school, and they did not want to interact with them. One girl's mother reported that a bully took her hearing aide, leaving her afraid to return to school. The siblings we interviewed did not mention bullying as being a concern. Most children with illnesses and their siblings (who also missed school to be at the hospital with the family) wanted to return to school, and reported missing their friends and "specials," such as art and physical education. They also missed participating in extracurricular activities.

Several issues were pertinent to homeschooling or the decision to homeschool. At times, it was "easier" to homeschool, because of many medical appointments and parental concerns that the school did not have the capabilities to manage the child's medical regimen. Medical issues inlcuded: needs for rest periods (issue of least complexity), modified assignments, needs to "not" carry books, required movement breaks, special diets, need for hydration, and administration of medicines (often multiple medicines at different time points during the day). Parents typically selected the curriculum for their child with an illness and siblings (who usually also were homeschooled), as some curricula could be expensive. For a few parents, the costs of medical care and even the gas to reach appointments often prohibited there being extra funds to afford homeschool curricula. School occurred when the child could concentrate (if the illness was taxing on energy levels) and when the parents could focus on delivering lessons. However, the parents who did purchase curricula were satisfied with the information and felt it met their children's needs. Other parents found their own lessons or developed curricula to match their children's interests. It was noteworthy that children participating in homeschooling were not receiving evaluations of their academic performance and abilities. Moreover, there were no regulations to determine rigor of the curricula being taught or to assess whether children were meeting academic markers for progress.

Limitations of the Current Evidence Base

Although there are many advances in the field to support children and families, there is still room to grow our knowledge. As such, there are several limitations to current knowledge that can be improved with further research. For instance, several of the studies we reviewed had small sample sizes. Others had larger sample sizes but included children with many types of illnesses across a broad age range. Consequently, it can be difficult to understand what works for whom, and more research across sites (in several hospitals or in different countries) could provide more information on the needs of specific groups. Interventions to enhance support and child and family functioning showed some positive outcomes, but results did vary across types of illness (Law et al., 2019). At the same time, it will be important to build the evidence base as there is not consistent evidence for some therapies, such as motivational interviewing, having a positive impact on child and parent outcomes. Improving quality of life for the child and their family is critical and measuring the impact of interventions on quality of life could be incorporated in studies, to determine broader impact of the interventions. It was noteworthy that studies did not always include long-term follow-up of child and family progress, and this would shed light on longevity of interventions. Long-term assessment of how the child and family are doing would also begin to tell us what types of interventions are needed at different phases of the child and family's journey in coping with difficulties, stress, as well as the waxing and waning course of the child's illness.

Conclusion

Children with chronic illnesses face unique challenges in maintaining school success during and after hospitalization. Evidence-based programs that support school success for these children are essential for ensuring that they continue to thrive academically, socially, and emotionally. Hospital-to-school reintegration programs, hospital school programs, psychological interventions, technology-assisted learning, peer and parent support programs, and therapeutic interventions play crucial roles in helping children overcome the barriers posed by chronic illness and hospitalization. By implementing these programs, we can provide the support necessary for children with chronic illnesses to succeed in school and lead fulfilling lives despite their health challenges.

It may be important to organize interventions to "match" interventions to problems typically faced by children with chronic illnesses. There is a model for this. Chorpita and Weisz (2009) developed the *MATCH-ADTC* (*MATCH-ADTC: Modular Approach to Therapy for Children with Anxiety, Depression, or Conduct Problems*) to create a modular approach to therapy for child mental health problems. It might be beneficial to develop a similar treatment approach (and manual) for assisting children and families in coping with chronic illnesses. Modules for therapeutic activities and action steps for improving academic achievement and management of the child's illness in the school setting could be developed. Furthermore, outlining steps for connecting children and parents to support groups and providing details about therapeutic interventions for children and parents (e.g., CBT and PS) could be provided in the manual. Our search did reveal one clinical trial, using the *MATCH-ADTC* to provide mental health interventions for youth with epilepsy (Bennett et al., 2021), and we believe using this approach for children with different types of illnesses is one way to provide knowledge of treatment approaches and advance treatment in the field. It may be advantageous to broaden information in the *MATCH-ADTC* (Chorpita & Weisz, 2009) or create a new manual like this one for professionals assisting children with chronic illnesses and their families. This would place valuable information at the fingertips of health care professionals. When addressing therapeutic interventions for children with chronic illnesses, it will be imperative to address interventions to improve school integration and emotional support of the child and family.

In sum, although the emotional and social challenges faced by children in the hospital are significant, there are a range of evidence-based interventions to help these children build resilience, enhance social connections, and develop effective coping strategies. Psychological interventions like CBT and problem-solving approaches as well as peer and parent support programs offer valuable support for hospitalized children. By addressing the emotional, social, and cognitive needs of children during their hospital stay, these interventions help children cope with the stress of illness and hospitalizations while fostering resilience. As research continues to explore and refine these interventions, comprehensive, developmentally appropriate, and evidence-based programs can play a crucial role in promoting the emotional well-being of children facing chronic illness and hospitalization.

Author Note. We would like to acknowledge Nneka Bonner and Joseph Lampton for their invaluable support and guidance.

References

Anthony, B. J., Serkin, C., Kahn, N., Troxel, M., & Shank, J. (2019). Tracking progress in peer-delivered family-to-family support. *Psychological Services, 16*(3), 388–401. https://doi.org/10.1037/ser0000256

Baker, K., & Claridge, A. M. (2023). "I have a Ph.D. in my daughter": Mother and child experiences of living with childhood chronic illness. *Journal of Child and Family Studies, 32*, 2625–2636. https://doi.org/10.1007/s10826-022-02506-8

Barnett, T., Goldfeld, S., & Kelaher, M. (2020). Evaluating the effectiveness of education support programs for hospitalized students with chronic health conditions: Protocol for a feasibility study of a controlled trial. *Continuity in Education, 1*(1), 126–135. https://doi.org/10.5334/cie.10

Barrio-Cortes, J., Benito-Sánchez, B., Sánchez-Ruano, R., García-Hernández, C. A., Beca-Martínez, M. T., Martínez-Cuevas, M., Castaño-Reguillo, A., & Muñoz-Lagos, C. (2024). Utilization of healthcare services in patients with chronic diseases under 18 years old: Differences and contributing factors. *Journal of Personalized Medicine, 14*(9), 956. https://doi.org/10.3390/jpm14090956

Bennett, S. D., Cross, J. H., Coughtrey, A. E., Heyman, I., Ford, T., Chorpita, B., Moss-Morris, R., Byford, S., Dalrymple, E., Reilly, C., Stephenson, T., Doré, C., Varadkar, S., Blackstone, J., Chowdhury, K., Ganguli, P., Deane, L., MICE Study Team, & Shafran, R. (2021). M.I.C.E-Mental Health Intervention for Children with Epilepsy: A randomised controlled, multi-centre clinical trial evaluating the clinical and cost-effectiveness of MATCH-ADTC in addition to usual care compared to usual care alone for children and young people with common mental health disorders and epilepsy-study protocol. *Trials, 22*(1), 132. https://doi.org/10.1186/s13063-020-05003-9

Boyd, J. R., & Hunsberger, M. (1998). Chronically ill children with repeated hospitalizations: Their perceptions and suggested interventions. *Journal of Pediatric Nursing, 13*(6), 330–342.

Caggiano, G., Brunetti, L. I. G., Ho, K., Piovani, A., & Quaranta, A. (2021). Hospital school program: The right to education for long-term care children. *International Journal of Environmental Research and Public Health, 18*(21), 11435. https://doi.org/10.3390/ijerph182111435

Canter, K. S., & Roberts, M. C. (2012). A systematic and quantitative review of interventions to facilitate school reentry for children with chronic health conditions. *Journal of Pediatric Psychology, 37*(10), 1065–1075. https://doi.org/10.1093/jpepsy/jss071

Carlton, E. F., Donnelly, J. P., Prescott, H. C., Asaro, L. A., Barbaro, R. P., Watson, R. S., Curley, M. A. Q., & RESTORE Study Investigators. (2021). School and work absences after critical care hospitalization for pediatric acute respiratory failure: A secondary analysis of a cluster randomized trial. *JAMA Network Open, 4*(12). https://doi.org/10.1001/jamanetworkopen.2021.40732

Catanzano, M., Bennett, S. D., Sanderson, C., Patel, M., Manzotti, G., Kerry, E., Coughtrey, A. E., Liang, H., Heyman, I., & Shafran, R. (2020). Brief psychological interventions for psychiatric disorders in young people with long term physical health conditions: A systematic review and meta-analysis. *Journal of Psychosomatic Research, 136*. https://doi.org/10.1016/j.jpsychores.2020.110187

Chin, J.-C., & Tsuei, M. (2014). A multi-modal digital game-based learning environment for hospitalized children with chronic illnesses. *Educational Technology & Society, 17*(4), 366–378. https://www.jstor.org/stable/jeductechsoci.17.4.366

Chorpita, B. F., & Weisz, J. R. (2009). *MATCH-ADTC: Modular approach to therapy for children with anxiety. Depression, trauma, or conduct problems*. PracticeWise.

Ciucci, E., Tomberli, L., Amore, E., Smorti, A., Maffei, F., & Vagnoli, L. (2024). The effects of hospital-based school lessons on children's emotions, distress and pain. *Continuity in Education, 5*(1), 100–110. https://doi.org/10.5334/cie.118

Cohn, L. N., Pechlivanoglou, P., Lee, Y., Mahant, S., Orkin, J., Marson, A., & Cohen, E. (2020). Health outcomes of parents of children with chronic illness: A systematic review and meta-analysis. *Journal of Pediatrics, 218*, 166–177.e2. https://doi.org/10.1016/j.jpeds.2019.10.068

Compas, B. E., Jaser, S. S., Dunn, M. J., & Rodriguez, E. M. (2012). Coping with chronic illness in childhood and adolescence. *Annual Review of Clinical Psychology, 8*, 455–450. https://doi.org/10.1146/annurev-clinpsy-032511-143108

Day, M., Clarke, S. A., Castillo-Eito, L., & Rowe, R. (2020). Psychoeducation for children with chronic conditions: A systematic review and meta-analysis. *Journal of Pediatric Psychology, 45*(4), 386–398. https://doi.org/10.1093/jpepsy/jsaa015

Di Padova, M., Pettoello-Mantovani, M., & Dipace, A. (2024). School in the hospital, the key role of an educating community. *Global Pediatrics, 9*. https://doi.org/10.1016/j.gpeds.2024.100204

Douma, M., Maurice-Stam, H., Gorter, B., Houtzager, B. A., Vreugdenhil, H. J. I., Waaldijk, M., Wiltink, L., Grootenhuis, M. A., & Scholten, L. (2021). Online psychosocial group intervention for adolescents with a chronic illness: A randomized controlled trial. *Internet Interventions, 26*. https://doi.org/10.1016/j.invent.2021.100447

Doupnik, S. K., Hill, D., Palakshappa, D., Worsley, D., Bae, H., Shaik, A., Qiu, M. K., Marsac, M., & Feudtner, C. (2017). Parent coping support interventions during acute pediatric hospitalizations: A meta-analysis. *Pediatrics, 140*(3). https://doi.org/10.1542/peds.2016-4171

Edwards, J., Waite-Jones, J., Schwarz, T., & Swallow, V. (2021). Digital technologies for children and parents sharing self-management in childhood chronic or long-term conditions: A scoping review. *Children (Basel, Switzerland), 8*(12). https://doi.org/10.3390/children8121203

Emerson, N. D., Distelberg, B., Morrell, H. E., Williams-Reade, J., Tapanes, D., & Montgomery, S. (2016). Quality of life and school absenteeism in children with chronic illness. *The Journal of School Nursing, 32*(4), 258–266. https://doi.org/10.1177/1059840515615401

Forrest, C. B., Koenigsberg, L. J., Eddy Harvey, F., Maltenfort, M. G., & Halfon, N. (2025). Trends in US children's mortality, chronic conditions, obesity, functional status, and symptoms. *JAMA, 334*(6), 509–516. https://doi.org/10.1001/jama.2025.9855

Guy-Evans, O. (2024). Bronfenbrenner's ecological systems theory. *Simply Psychology*. www.simplypsychology.org/bronfenbrenner.html#Classroom-Application

Harden, C., Rea, H., Buchanan-Perry, I., Gee, B., & Johnson, A. (2020). A multidisciplinary educational approach for children with chronic illness: An intervention case study. *Continuity in Education, 1*(1), 8–21. https://doi.org/10.5334/cie.2

Helms, A. S., Schmiegelow, K., Brok, J., Johansen, C., Thorsteinsson, T., Simovska, V., & Larsen, H. B. (2016). Facilitation of school re-entry and peer acceptance of children with cancer: A review and meta-analysis of intervention studies. *European Journal of Cancer Care, 25*(1), 170–179. https://doi.org/10.1111/ecc.12230

Hill, E. L., Reifschneider, K., Ramsing, R., Turnage, M., & Goff, J. (2019). Family diabetes camp: Fostering resiliency among campers and parents. *Diabetes Spectrum, 32*(2), 86–92. https://doi.org/10.2337/ds18-0001

Hu, N., Fardell, J., Wakefield, C. E., Marshall, G. M., Bell, J. C., Nassar, N., & Lingam, R. (2022). School academic performance of children hospitalised with a chronic condition. *Archives of Disease in Childhood, 107*(3), 289–296. https://doi.org/10.1136/archdischild-2020-321285

Individuals with Disabilities Education Act. Amendments of 2004, Public Law 105-17, 20 U.S.C. 1400 et. Seq. (2004).

Kassab, S., & Claybourn, C. (2023). 504 plans versus IEP: A guide for parents. *U.S. News and World Report*. https://www.usnews.com/education/k12/articles/504-plan-versus-iep-a-guide-for-parents

Kirk, S., & Milnes, L. J. (2021). Peer support for young people with chronic conditions. In J. N. T. Sattoe, A. van Staa, & S. R. Hilberink (Eds.), *Self-management of young people with chronic conditions: A strength-based approach for empowerment and support* (pp. 135–160). Springer Nature Switzerland AG. https://doi.org/10.1007/978-3-030-64293-8_7

Kohl, S. E., & Barnett, E. D. (2020). What do we know about travel for children with special health care needs? A review of the literature. *Travel Medicine and Infectious Disease, 34*, 101438. https://doi.org/10.1016/j.tmaid.2019.06.009

Koumarianou, A., Symeonidi, A. E., Kattamis, A., Linardatou, K., Chrousos, G. P., & Darviri, C. (2021). A review of psychosocial interventions targeting families of children with cancer. *Palliative & Supportive Care, 19*(1), 103–118. https://doi.org/10.1017/S1478951520000449

Kratchman, A., Barkman, D., Conaboy, K., de la Motte, A., Biblow, R., & Bevans, K. (2015). The children's Hospital of Philadelphia Family Partners Program: Promoting child and family-centered care in pediatrics. *Patient Experience Journal, 2*(1), 50–60. https://doi.org/10.35680/2372-0247.1063

Kvarnström, K., Westerholm, A., Airaksinen, M., & Liira, H. (2021). Factors contributing to medication adherence in patients with a chronic condition: A scoping review of qualitative research. *Pharmaceutics, 13*(7), 1100. https://doi.org/10.3390/pharmaceutics13071100

Lancaster, K., Bhopti, A., Kern, M. L., Taylor, R., Janson, A., & Harding, K. (2023). Effectiveness of peer support programmes for improving well-being and quality of life in parents/carers of children with disability or chronic illness: A systematic review. *Child: Care, Health and Development, 49*(3), 485–496. https://doi.org/10.1111/cch.13063

Law, E., Fisher, E., Eccleston, C., & Palermo, T. M. (2019). Psychological interventions for parents of children and adolescents with chronic illness. *The Cochrane Database of Systematic Reviews, 3*(3), CD009660. https://doi.org/10.1002/14651858.CD009660.pub4

Leite, A. C. A. B., Rodrigues, A. L., Alvarenga, W. A., Polita, N. B., Silva-Rodrigues, F. M., Bolis, L. O., Meherali, S., & Nascimento, L. C. (2023). School reintegration of children and adolescents with chronic illness from the mothers' perspective: A qualitative study. *Child: Care, Health and Development, 49*(1), 181–188. https://doi.org/10.1111/cch.13031

Lewis, P., Klineberg, E., Towns, S., Moore, K., & Steinbeck, K. (2016). The effects of introducing peer support to young people with a chronic illness. *Journal of Child and Family Studies, 25*, 2541–2553. https://doi.org/10.1007/s10826-016-0427-4

Lum, A., Wakefield, C. E., Donnan, B., Burns, M. A., Fardell, J. E., Jaffe, A., Kasparian, N. A., Kennedy, S. E., Leach, S. T., Lemberg, D. A., & Marshall, G. M. (2019). School students with chronic illness have unmet academic, social, and emotional school needs. *School Psychology, 34*(6), 627–636. https://doi-org.uc.idm.oclc.org/10.1037/spq0000311

Marshall, K. H., Pincus, H. A., Tesson, S., Lingam, R., Woolfenden, S. R., & Kasparian, N. A. (2022). Integrated psychological care in pediatric hospital settings for children with complex chronic illness and their families: A systematic review. *Psychology & Health, 39*(4), 452–478. https://doi.org/10.1080/08870446.2022.2072843

Matthews, K. D. (2024). General and special education teacher experiences and support strategies for adolescent students experiencing chronic health conditions. *Walden Dissertations and Doctoral Studies*. 15659. https://scholarworks.waldenu.edu/dissertations/15659

McCabe, E. M., Kaskoun, J. R., & Strauss, S. M. (2021). School nurses as vital members of 504 and individualized educational program teams: Do district-level policies make a difference in school nurses' involvement? *Policy, Politics & Nursing Practice, 22*(3), 191–200. https://doi.org/10.1177/15271544211011959

Merianos, A. L., Vidourek, R. A., King, K. A., & Nabors, L. (2015). Hospital, school, and community-based strategies to enhance the quality of life of youth with chronic illnesses. *Applied Research Quality Life, 10*, 329–342. https://doi.org/10.1007/s11482-014-9311-9

Merianos, A. L., King, K. A., Vidourek, R. A., & Nabors, L. A. (2016). Mentoring and peer-led interventions to improve quality of life outcomes among adolescents with chronic illnesses. *Applied Research Quality Life, 11*, 1009–1023. https://doi.org/10.1007/s11482-015-9415-x

Mokkink, L. B., van der Lee, J. H., Grootenhuis, M. A., Offringa, M., Heymans, H. S., & Dutch. National Consensus Committee Chronic Diseases and Health Conditions in Childhood. (2008). Defining chronic diseases and health conditions in childhood (0-18 years of age): National consensus in The Netherlands. *European Journal of Pediatrics, 167*(12), 1441–1447. https://doi.org/10.1007/s00431-008-0697-y

Nabbijohn, A. N., Tomlinson, R. M., Lee, S., Morrongiello, B. A., & McMurtry, C. M. (2021). The measurement and conceptualization of coping responses in pediatric chronic pain populations: A scoping review. *Frontiers in Psychology, 12*, 680277. https://doi.org/10.3389/fpsyg.2021.680277

Naset.org home page. NASET News Alert RSS. (2008). https://www.naset.org/professional-resources/exceptional-students-and-disability-information/other-health-impairments/comprehensive-overview-of-other-health-impairments

Nationwide Children's. (2025). Connecting families. *Nationwide Children's Hospital*. www.nationwidechildrens.org/family-resources-education/patient-and-family-centered-care/connecting-families

Olsson, C. A., Boyce, M. F., Toumbourou, J. W., & Sawyer, S. M. (2005). The role of peer support in facilitating psychosocial adjustment to chronic illness in adolescence. *Clinical Child Psychology and Psychiatry, 10*(1), 78–87. https://doi.org/10.1177/1359104505048793

Psihogios, A. M., Fellmeth, H., Schwartz, L. A., & Barakat, L. P. (2019). Family functioning and medical adherence across children and adolescents with chronic health conditions: A meta-analysis. *Journal of Pediatric Psychology, 44*(1), 84–97. https://doi.org/10.1093/jpepsy/jsy044

Rohan, J. M., & Verma, T. (2020). Psychological considerations in pediatric chronic illness: Case examples. *International Journal of Environmental Research and Public Health, 17*(5), 1644. https://doi.org/10.3390/ijerph17051644

Rolland, J. S. (1987). Chronic illness and the life cycle: A conceptual framework. *Family Process, 26*, 203–211.

Sansom-Daly, U. M., Peate, M., Wakefield, C. E., Bryant, R. A., & Cohn, R. J. (2012). A systematic review of psychological interventions for adolescents and young adults living with chronic illness. *Health Psychology, 31*(3), 380–393. https://doi.org/10.1037/a0025977

Sattoe, J. N., Bal, M. I., Roelofs, P. D., Bal, R., Miedema, H. S., & van Staa, A. (2015). Self-management interventions for young people with chronic conditions: A systematic overview. *Patient Education and Counseling, 98*(6), 704–715. https://doi.org/10.1016/j.pec.2015.03.004

Schultz, S. (2020). Differences between a 504 plan and an individualized education program (IEP). *National Education Association.* https://www.nea.org/professional-excellence/student-engagement/tools-tips/differences-between-504-plan-and-individualized-education-program-iep

Shaw, S. R., & McCabe, P. C. (2008). Hospital-to-school transition for children with chronic illness: Meeting the new challenges of an evolving health care system. *Psychology in the Schools, 45*(1), 74–87. https://doi.org/10.1002/pits.20280

Spiel, C. F., Evans, S. W., & Langberg, J. M. (2014). Evaluating the content of individualized education programs and 504 plans of young adolescents with attention deficit/hyperactivity disorder. *School Psychology Quarterly, 29*(4), 452–468. https://doi.org/10.1037/spq0000101

Steinke, S. M., Elam, M., Irwin, M. K., Sexton, K., & McGraw, A. (2016). Pediatric hospital school programming: An examination of educational services for students who are hospitalized. *Physical Disabilities: Education and Related Services, 35*(1), 28–45. https://doi.org/10.14434/pders.v35i1.20896

Thabrew, H., Stasiak, K., Hetrick, S. E., Wong, S., Huss, J. H., & Merry, S. N. (2018). E-health interventions for anxiety and depression in children and adolescents with long-term physical conditions. *The. Cochrane Database of Systematic Reviews, 8*(8), CD012489. https://doi.org/10.1002/14651858.CD012489.pub2

U.S. Department of Education, Office of Special Education Programs. (2006). IDEA Regulations: Individualized Education Program (IEP). [34 CFR 300.320(c)] [20 U.S.C. 1414(d)(1)(A)(i)(VIII)(cc)] https://sites.ed.gov/idea/files/IEP_10-4-06.pdf

Wazevich, M., Bonner, N., Lampton, J., Justice, R., & Nabors, L. (2024, October). *Child and parent perspectives of "school out of school" at a Ronald McDonald House for children with chronic illnesses and their siblings.* Paper presentation at the American Public Health Association Conference: Minneapolis, MN.

Wiemann, C. M., Graham, S. C., Garland, B. H., Hergenroeder, A. C., Raphael, J. L., Sanchez-Fournier, B. E., Benavides, J. M., & Warren, L. J. (2019). Development of a group-based, peer-mentor intervention to promote disease self-management skills among youth with chronic medical conditions. *Journal of Pediatric Nursing, 48,* 1–9. https://doi.org/10.1016/j.pedn.2019.05.013

Wijlaars, L. P., Gilbert, R., & Hardelid, P. (2016). Chronic conditions in children and young people: Learning from administrative data. *Archives of Disease in Childhood, 101*(10), 881–885. https://doi.org/10.1136/archdischild-2016-310716

Wikel, K., & Markelz, A. M. (2023). Chronic health conditions, school attendance, and socioeconomic factors: A literature review. *Journal of Special Education Apprenticeship, 12*(2), Article 9. https://doi.org/10.58729/2167-3454.1173

Wodinski, L. M., Mattson McCrady, H. M., Oswald, C. M., Lyste, N. J. M., & Forbes, K. L. L. (2017). Family bedside orientations: An innovative peer support model to enhance a culture of family-centered care at the Stollery Children's Hospital. *Paediatrics & Child Health., 22*(7), 387–390. https://doi.org/10.1093/pch/pxx117

Chapter 10
Navigating the System as a Family of a Child with a Developmental Disability or Health Condition

Kara B. Ayers, Jocelyn Gomez, and Stephanie Weber

Abstract This chapter explores the challenges faced by families of children with developmental disabilities or health conditions as they navigate fragmented support systems across medical, educational, social, and community services. It highlights the crucial roles played by care navigators, case managers, family navigators, and disability advocates, emphasizing how their coordinated efforts can ease family burdens and enhance well-being. Using interdisciplinary care models and visual service maps, the chapter shows how collaboration reduces redundancies, aligns therapy and educational goals, and adapts to family needs—an approach proven especially vital during the COVID-19 pandemic. The authors critique traditional system-focused metrics and advocate for family-centered outcomes, such as children's participation in valued activities and families' ability to manage responsibilities, measured through both quantitative and qualitative feedback. The chapter calls for routine inclusion of family voices in policy, integrated funding, and efforts to reduce inequities. Ultimately, it argues for service integration that supports everyday family life and child development, grounded in families' lived experiences.

Keywords Children with developmental disabilities · Services; educational support services · Care coordination systems · Support networks · Effective communication systems · Family-driven innovations

K. B. Ayers (✉) · S. Weber
Division of Developmental and Behavioral Pediatrics, Cincinnati Children's Hospital Medical Center, Cincinnati, OH, USA
e-mail: kara.ayers@cchmc.org

College of Medicine, University of Cincinnati, Cincinnati, OH, USA

J. Gomez
Department of Pediatrics, Baylor College of Medicine, Houston, TX, USA

Texas Children's Hospital, Houston, TX, USA

L. Nabors and T. Stanton-Chapman (eds.), *Developmental Disabilities and Chronic Illness in Young Children*, Springer Series on Child and Family Studies,
https://doi.org/10.1007/978-3-032-08523-8_10

Families of children with developmental disabilities and chronic health conditions face complex challenges in navigating multiple service systems and support networks. The landscape of available services spans medical care, educational support, therapeutic interventions, and community-based resources. While these services aim to promote child development and family wellbeing, accessing and coordinating them often requires significant time, knowledge, and persistence from families who are already managing complex care needs (Kuo et al., 2018; Luke et al., 2020).

Consider Justine's family: Her 8-year-old son, David, has cerebral palsy and attends weekly physical therapy, occupational therapy, and speech therapy. Justine, who uses a wheelchair herself, must coordinate these services around her other children's schedules while managing her own healthcare needs. A typical week involves juggling three different therapy appointments at two different locations, communicating with five healthcare providers, occasionally attending IEP meetings at school, and ensuring proper documentation reaches everyone involved in David's care. When David's wheelchair needs repairs, Justine must coordinate with both the equipment vendor and insurance company while finding alternative transportation to maintain his therapy schedule. This intricate dance of coordination occurs against the backdrop of everyday family life—work, meals, homework, and family time.

The journey through these systems can be particularly challenging for families facing additional barriers related to language, culture, disability status, geographic location, or socioeconomic circumstances (Pankewicz et al., 2020). Parents and caregivers—including those with disabilities themselves—must often serve as both advocates and care coordinators while balancing the needs of their entire family. Understanding this reality is essential for developing more equitable, accessible, and family-centered approaches to service delivery.

Types of Services and Support Systems

Medical and Healthcare Services

The foundation of support typically begins with medical and healthcare services, encompassing primary care providers, medical specialists, hospitals, and community health clinics. For many families, this includes coordinating care between multiple providers while ensuring communication flows effectively across the healthcare team (Kuo et al., 2018). Critical to this process is the establishment of a medical home—a model of primary care that is accessible, continuous, comprehensive, family-centered, coordinated, compassionate, and culturally effective (Council on Children with Disabilities and Medical Home Implementation Project Advisory Committee et al., 2014).

Educational Support Services

Educational services form another crucial pillar, including special education programs, individualized education plans (IEPs), and school-based therapies. These services require careful coordination between families, educators, school-based and hospital-based healthcare providers to ensure alignment with the child's medical needs and developmental goals. The intersection of medical and educational services often presents particular challenges, especially for families navigating both systems simultaneously (Kuo et al., 2018). In some cases, services simply do not exist to meet the needs of families. There are exceptionally limited childcare options for children with complex medical needs. Childcare facilities are not required to accept or accommodate needs and most are not staffed to care for children with feeding tubes and other medical devices. Many parents must leave the workforce because there are no childcare options for their children with disabilities (Whitmore et al., 2023).

Despite decades of research clearly indicating the benefits of inclusive educational placements for children with disabilities, the state of inclusion in schools in the United States still falters (Wehmeyer et al., 2021). Parents are described as "equal partners" in the IEP process but there are few opportunities to learn what supports are available in schools, how to advocate for them, and what to do if they are denied (Lanchak et al., 2024).

Developmental and Therapeutic Services

Children with developmental disabilities often need access to various therapeutic interventions, including:

- Speech and language therapy
- Occupational therapy
- Physical therapy
- Behavioral interventions
- Mental health services

These services may be provided through early intervention programs, school systems, medical facilities, or private practices, requiring families to coordinate across multiple providers and settings (Sheppard & Moran, 2022). While parents value access to these services, they also desire access to community connections, leisure activities, and social activities for their children. Difficulty finding and coordinating information about these opportunities is a significant barrier for families (Lanchak et al., 2024).

Community Support Programs

Community-based supports play a vital role in addressing the holistic needs of children and families. These may include:

- Family support networks and peer mentoring
- Respite care services
- Transportation assistance
- Recreation programs
- Faith-based or cultural organizations
- Food security programs
- Housing assistance

The availability and accessibility of these programs often vary significantly based on geographic location and community resources. Too often, these community-based supports are seen as ancillary. A 2024 study on parent perspectives on navigating disability-related information and resources found, "Parents wanted their children (with disabilities) to experience an array of formative experiences" (Lanchak et al., 2024, p. 459). Parents' familiarity with local and community resources varied widely and was often limited—a problem compounded by the fact that even providers, including social workers and care coordinators, frequently lack comprehensive knowledge of available resources (Lanchak et al., 2024). This knowledge gap among professionals underscores the importance of partnering with disabled adults and families who often possess deep understanding of community resources and informal support networks that might not be apparent to traditional service providers. Research indicates that families of children with disabilities from marginalized communities, including those living in poverty or rural areas, face disproportionate barriers in accessing these vital support services (Pankewicz et al., 2020).

These barriers stem from multiple interconnected factors: geographic isolation limits access to specialized services and transportation options (Emerson & Llewellyn, 2021; Children's Hospital Association, 2021); economic constraints restrict families' abilities to afford services, take time off work, or travel to appointments (Parish & Thomas, 2022; Family Voices, 2023; systemic inequities in service distribution often leave underserved communities with fewer available resources (Zuckerman et al., 2021; National Council on Disability, 2023); and cultural or linguistic differences can create communication barriers between families and service providers (Magaña et al., 2021). Additionally, complex bureaucratic processes and eligibility requirements may be particularly challenging for families with limited educational resources or English proficiency to navigate (Musumeci & Rudowitz, 2022).

Care Coordination Systems

Given the complexity of navigating multiple service systems, care coordination has emerged as a critical component for supporting families (Family Voices, 2023). Effective care coordination is patient- and family-centered, assessment-driven, and team-based, designed to enhance both care delivery and family caregiving capabilities. This approach recognizes that families are the constant in their children's lives and must be empowered as full partners in the care coordination process (Antonelli et al., 2009; Musumeci & Rudowitz, 2022).

The success of care coordination efforts often depends on several key factors (Council on Children with Disabilities and Medical Home Implementation Project Advisory Committee et al., 2014):

- Clear communication channels between all providers and family members
- Respect for family expertise and preferences
- Cultural competency in service delivery
- Recognition of social determinants of health (Pankewicz et al., 2020)
- Flexible and responsive support systems (Nageswaran et al., 2024)
- Integration of services across different sectors (Gall et al., 2022)

Understanding these various systems and their interconnections is essential for both providers and families as they work together to create comprehensive, coordinated care plans that support optimal child development and family wellbeing. In the wake of the COVID-19 pandemic, the flexibility of care models has been increasingly relevant, including the use of telehealth and remote monitoring services, reducing the burden on families to frequently travel to various physical locations for care (Nageswaran et al., 2024).

Strategies for Successful Service Navigation

Building a Strong Support Network

The foundation of successful navigation begins with building a robust support network. Families need a multidisciplinary team to effectively navigate healthcare, education, and social systems. This network typically includes healthcare providers, social workers, care navigators, therapists, case managers, and educators working in concert to support the child and family's needs (Kuo et al., 2018). Some hospitals have recognized the critical intersection between healthcare and education by establishing school liaison positions—specialists who help families navigate educational systems and advocate for appropriate accommodations through 504 plans or IEPs (Individual Education Plans; Thibodaux et al., 2024). While these dedicated educational liaisons remain rare in healthcare settings, their success demonstrates the value of cross-system coordination (Frye et al., 2024). Programs like NaviCare/

SoinsNavi demonstrate how patient navigators can help families assemble, coordinate, and work effectively with their service teams (Doucet et al., 2019). The medical home framework, first outlined by the American Academy of Pediatrics in 2014 and then reaffirmed in April 2023, further emphasizes the importance of integrating primary care physicians, specialists, therapists, and community professionals into a cohesive team providing comprehensive care (Council on Children with Disabilities and Medical Home Implementation Project Advisory Committee et al., 2014).

Notably absent from many families' support networks are adults with disabilities who themselves have extensive experience navigating service systems. These individuals possess invaluable firsthand knowledge of both system navigation and the lived experience of disability, yet this potentially powerful resource remains largely untapped. Adults with disabilities could offer unique insights into effective advocacy strategies, share practical solutions for common barriers, and provide mentorship based on lived experience. Their expertise could be particularly valuable in helping families understand how to promote their child's autonomy and self-advocacy while navigating complex systems. Additionally, disabled adults often have deep knowledge of community resources and informal support networks that might not be apparent to traditional service providers. Some adults with disabilities share this navigational knowledge through social media, reaching audiences comprised of other adults with disabilities and parents of children with disabilities (Sweet et al., 2020). Healthcare systems and support organizations could enhance their services by intentionally incorporating disabled adults as peer mentors, advisors, or navigation specialists. This disconnect currently represents a missed opportunity for meaningful peer support and mentorship that could benefit both families and children (Cairncross, 2019).

Effective Communication Channels are Critical for Reducing Care Fragmentation

Effective communication channels are critical for reducing care fragmentation and ensuring shared understanding among team members. Many families report that communication gaps represent a significant challenge in their care journey, highlighting the essential role of case managers and care coordinators in bridging these gaps (Family Voices, 2023). Shared Plans of Care (SPoC) have emerged as valuable tools for ensuring information flows effectively among all providers while staying aligned with family goals and priorities (McAllister et al., 2018).

Creating collaborative partnerships between families, providers, and systems—such as healthcare, education, mental health, and social services—is another crucial element of successful navigation for children with disabilities. These systems often operate separately, each with their own language, eligibility requirements, and organizational structures, which can overwhelm families trying to access coordinated care. When families are meaningfully included in care design, it not only increases trust but ensures services align with family priorities, cultural values, and lived experiences. Innovative approaches like co-located services—such as school-based health programs—can facilitate stronger collaboration among stakeholders while making services more accessible to families (Currie et al., 2023).

Developing Advocacy Skills

Successful navigation requires families to develop strong advocacy skills. Understanding rights and entitlements under frameworks such as the Individuals with Disabilities Education Act (IDEA) and Americans with Disabilities Act (ADA) is fundamental. Many families benefit from education and advocacy programs that enhance their ability to advocate effectively for needed services. Care navigators and case managers often play a crucial role in helping families understand their legal protections and options for accessing services.

Documentation and record-keeping form another critical component of effective advocacy. Families must maintain accessible records of medical information, educational plans (IEPs/504 plans), therapy reports, and service timelines. While hospitals and insurance companies may provide their own case managers, families sometimes need to independently seek additional community-based support to help manage this documentation burden. Care coordination programs increasingly integrate documentation support into their services, often utilizing Shared Plans of Care to provide families with centralized records of care plans and service alignment (McAllister et al., 2018). However, the fragmentation of case management services means families may need to actively seek out and combine support from multiple sources to meet their comprehensive needs.

Learning to communicate effectively with providers represents a key advocacy skill that often develops over time (Szlamka et al., 2022). Families must learn to articulate their child's needs clearly and assertively to providers—a skill that can be particularly challenging when managing multiple providers or navigating complex healthcare systems. Parent training programs and navigation services increasingly emphasize building communication confidence, recognizing its importance in securing appropriate services and supports (Lanchak et al., 2024).

Coordinating Care Across Systems

Successful navigation requires strategic coordination across multiple systems. Integrated care planning helps document shared goals, roles, and responsibilities across all providers and systems involved in the child's care. Shared Plans of Care create structured strategies that integrate family priorities with system-specific goals, helping reduce duplication of efforts and aligning services across healthcare, education, and therapy sectors (McAllister et al., 2018).

Managing transitions between services presents particular challenges due to limited inter-system communication and varying eligibility criteria. Critical transition points—such as moving from early intervention to school-based systems or from pediatric to adult care—require careful planning and coordination. While there are multiple professionals who fulfill supportive roles to facilitate transition, the boundaries between their responsibilities can be confusing (see Table 10.1). Successful programs emphasize communication between providers and transition planning as an explicit care goal, ensuring continuity of services during these critical junctures (Kuo et al., 2018).

To illustrate how effective integration can work, consider a well-designed interdisciplinary medical setting: A child visits their primary care provider for a routine appointment, where standardized screening reveals concerns about food insecurity and behavioral challenges. Rather than simply making referrals, the provider directly connects with the clinic's social worker to address the family's immediate needs. The social worker, working alongside a case manager, helps the family access food assistance programs while a behavioral health specialist, embedded within the practice, provides immediate consultation. Simultaneously, the clinic's school liaison begins working with the family to ensure appropriate educational support is in place. This integrated approach means families receive comprehensive support without having to navigate multiple systems independently.

The challenge of information sharing across providers remains significant, with information silos between healthcare, educational, and community systems often disadvantaging families (Lanchak et al., 2024). Insurance barriers also frequently complicate families' efforts to access needed care, as inadequate or inconsistent

Table 10.1 Definitions of common roles in care coordination

Type of professional	Focus	Key duties
Care navigators	Medical	Healthcare professionals and sometimes peers (parents and other caregivers) who assist families in coordinating medical appointments, connecting them to resources, and navigating insurance and social services, typically working alongside primary care physicians.
Case managers	Broader social services	Professionals who help families assess needs, access resources, and navigate social service systems across multiple sectors to improve family wellbeing.
Family navigators	Caregiver focus	Peers to patients and their families who help relative caregivers (such as parents, grandparents, or other family members) access resources, understand their rights, and navigate support systems when raising children in their care.
Disability advocates	Focus on person or people with disabilities	People with disabilities who use their lived experience and systems knowledge to support other disabled people in navigating healthcare, education, and community services while promoting autonomy and self-determination.

coverage can delay or prevent access to essential services for children with disabilities (Houtrow et al., 2025). While innovations in centralized navigation centers and care integration frameworks are beginning to address these challenges through standardized communication tools and centralized information-sharing capabilities, such comprehensive models remain rare. Most families must still piece together services across disconnected systems, highlighting the need for broader adoption of integrated care approaches. Building effective navigation strategies requires attention to these interconnected elements while recognizing that each family's journey is unique. Success often depends on establishing strong collaborative relationships, developing effective advocacy skills, and implementing systematic approaches to care coordination—all while keeping family needs and preferences at the center of the process (Currie et al., 2023).

Evaluating and Adjusting Service Integration

The complexity of coordinating services across health care, educational, and community systems arises from differences in eligibility criteria, organizational structures, and communication norms, requiring families and providers to adapt continually as needs and circumstances change (Family Voices, 2023). As children's situations evolve, regular evaluation and timely adjustments are necessary to address gaps, eliminate redundancies, and respond flexibly to new challenges or changes in family goals. Effective care coordination thus relies on systematic feedback from families, ongoing assessment of system performance, and proactive modification of strategies to ensure truly family-centered, integrated support.

Family-Centered Assessment of Care Coordination

Traditional approaches to measuring service effectiveness often focus too narrowly on individual service outcomes rather than evaluating how well services work together as an integrated system. For instance, a speech therapy program might track specific communication goals, while an occupational therapy program measures fine motor skills, but neither evaluates how these services complement each other or fit into the family's daily routine. Care mapping has emerged as a powerful tool for families and providers to visualize and assess the current state of service integration (Adams et al., 2019). Figure 10.1, which was adapted from Kuo et al. (2018), presents an example of care mapping. This type of visual representation helps identify gaps, redundancies, and opportunities for better coordination while centering the family's experience.

Figure 10.1 presents a care map for Max, age 17, and this map illustrates the interconnected systems and supports in his life, including medical care, educational services, family support networks, leisure activities, and financial considerations. The star at the center shows Max surrounded by family members (Mom, Dad, Ava, and Grace). This care map is adapted from a model shared by Kuo et al. (2018), but

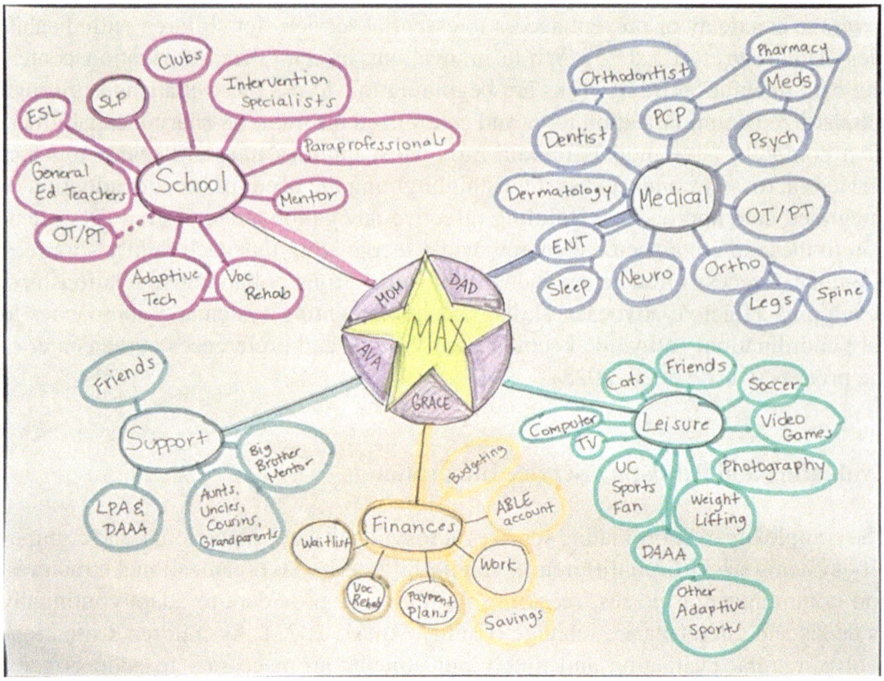

Fig. 10.1 Sample care map

names have been changed to protect privacy. This visualization exercise provides an opportunity for care coordinators and navigators to support a family and transitioning youth with disabilities to reorganize their care plan with increased focus on individual and family priorities. Through this process, redundancies, excessive appointments, and medical bills can be decreased, while making more room for recreation, leisure, health, and well-being.

Consider a family whose child receives both school-based and private therapies. While each service might report progress on individual goals, the family's measure of success often centers on practical outcomes: Has coordination between providers reduced the number of times they need to leave work for appointments? Are therapy goals aligned to support their child's participation in valued family and community activities? Are providers sharing information effectively, or does the family still need to repeatedly relay the same updates? These real-world measures of integration effectiveness often matter more to families than traditional clinical metrics. Mapping all the services a child and family interact with—sometimes called a "service map" or "care coordination map"—can help identify gaps, redundancies, or missed opportunities for collaboration. Implementing changes based on these maps, such as connecting providers directly or establishing shared goals, can improve service integration and ensure care is more responsive to family priorities (Family Voices, 2023; Kuo et al., 2020).

Identifying Need for Adjustments

Service needs naturally evolve as children develop and family circumstances change. A child who initially needed intensive physical therapy might develop new social or communication goals as they enter school. A family's ability to coordinate morning therapy appointments might shift when a parent's work schedule changes. Yet families often encounter rigid systems that resist modification, forcing them to maintain service schedules and approaches that no longer serve their needs effectively (Nageswaran et al., 2024).

The rigidity of service systems particularly impacts families from marginalized communities who may already be navigating additional systemic barriers (Emerson & Llewellyn, 2021). For example, a family living in a rural area might struggle to adjust therapy schedules when transportation assistance programs have inflexible hours. A family whose primary language isn't English faces compounded challenges: not only are there communication barriers when trying to modify services across multiple providers, but essential resources and follow-up recommendations are often provided only in English. This failure to provide linguistically appropriate materials means families cannot access crucial information about their child's care, forcing them to rely on individual providers' willingness to assist with translation and service coordination (Pankewicz et al., 2020).

Implementing Changes

The process of implementing changes often reveals the fragmentation inherent in disability service systems. A family seeking to adjust their child's therapy schedule to accommodate a new school program might need to coordinate with multiple providers, navigate different administrative processes, and ensure all team members understand and support the changes. Some innovative programs are developing more responsive approaches, such as regular multi-team review meetings or shared electronic platforms where updates can be communicated to all providers simultaneously (Altman et al., 2018; Gall et al., 2022). What sets these approaches apart is their emphasis on real-time, bidirectional communication and family engagement, which reduce delays and miscommunication. By creating centralized points of information exchange and decision-making, they streamline coordination and promote collective accountability among providers. This not only lightens the navigation burden on families but also ensures care adjustments are timely, coherent, and truly reflective of the child's evolving needs. These approaches recognize that families shouldn't have to navigate multiple bureaucracies to make simple adjustments to their service plans.

The COVID-19 pandemic forced many systems to demonstrate greater flexibility than previously thought possible. The rapid adoption of telehealth services showed that systems can evolve when properly motivated. Some families found that virtual options actually improved service integration by reducing travel time and making it easier to coordinate care across providers; These experiences highlight how system flexibility can enhance rather than compromise service quality (Nageswaran et al., 2024).

Measuring Impact

Evaluating the impact of service integration requires attention to outcomes that matter to families but are often overlooked by traditional metrics. While providers might focus on specific developmental achievements, families often measure success by their child's ability to participate fully in family life, develop meaningful relationships, and engage in their community. A service integration plan might be considered successful when a family can attend their child's therapy sessions without sacrificing their other children's activities, or when they can take a family vacation without extensive coordination between multiple providers. Best practice in assessing impact includes incorporating family-reported outcome measures and regular qualitative feedback to capture how well services reduce daily burdens and support family priorities beyond clinical goals.

The disconnect between system-centered and family-centered measures of success highlights the ongoing need for more holistic approaches to evaluation. When systems prioritize administrative efficiency over family experience, they risk creating technically proficient but practically ineffective service plans. True success in service integration should be measured by how well it supports both child development and family wellbeing, recognizing that these goals are inextricably linked. A holistic evaluation should incorporate multiple steps, including gathering quantitative data on developmental progress alongside qualitative feedback from families about their lived experiences and daily challenges. This process involves regular check-ins with families to assess satisfaction, identify unmet needs, and adjust services accordingly. Additionally, coordination among providers to share information and jointly review outcomes helps ensure that evaluation reflects the full context of the child's life and family dynamics, enabling continuous, adaptive improvements that align with family priorities.

Future Directions and Recommendations

The landscape of service delivery for children with developmental disabilities continues to evolve, shaped by technological advances, changing family needs, and lessons learned from system failures. While the COVID-19 pandemic exposed significant gaps in service systems, it also accelerated adoption of innovative approaches that may benefit families long-term (Fong et al., 2023; Nageswaran et al., 2024).

Emerging Trends in Service Delivery

Technology integration has transformed how families can access and coordinate services, though not always equitably. Virtual platforms for care coordination show promise in reducing the burden of multiple appointments and improving communication between providers (Fong et al., 2023). However, the digital divide remains a significant concern, particularly for families in rural areas or those with limited technological resources (Lanchak et al., 2024). The rapid expansion of telehealth during the pandemic demonstrated both its potential and limitations. While some families found virtual services more accessible and easier to coordinate, others struggled with the loss of hands-on therapeutic interactions. Future service models will likely need to balance virtual and in-person options, allowing families to choose what works best for their circumstances (Fong et al., 2023; Nageswaran et al., 2024).

Perhaps most promising are family-driven innovations emerging from communities themselves. Social media platforms have become powerful tools for sharing navigational knowledge, with disabled adults and parents creating informal but effective information networks (Sweet et al., 2020). These grassroots efforts often prove more responsive to family needs than traditional service systems.

Policy Implications and Advocacy Priorities

System reform opportunities must address fundamental inequities in service access and coordination. This includes:

- Developing policies that recognize and compensate families for care coordination labor
- Creating funding mechanisms that support integrated service delivery
- Establishing standards for cross-system communication and collaboration
- Requiring meaningful inclusion of disabled adults and families in policy development

The shift toward value-based care presents opportunities to reimagine how services are funded and delivered. Payment models must evolve to support comprehensive care coordination rather than fragmenting services based on funding streams. This includes recognizing that community participation and family wellbeing are essential outcomes worthy of support (Gall et al., 2022; Kuo et al., 2018). Community participation can mean enabling children with disabilities to join recreation programs, participate in after-school clubs, or attend local events, while family support may include connecting parents to peer support groups, respite care, and resources that help all family members thrive. By investing in services that foster these connections—such as transportation to community activities or funding for family-led support networks—value-based approaches ensure that care extends beyond clinical settings to promote true inclusion and holistic wellbeing for families.

Building Sustainable Solutions

Creating sustainable improvements in service systems requires attention to both evidence-based practices and family wisdom. Consider a children's hospital that transformed its service delivery model by partnering with local families and disabled adults to redesign their care coordination program. Instead of measuring success solely through clinical outcomes, they developed metrics that reflected family priorities: reduced waiting times between appointments, decreased paperwork burden, and improved access to community activities. The center also created a family advisory committee that includes disabled adults from the community, ensuring that program improvements reflect real experiences and needs.

This example demonstrates how sustainable solutions emerge when systems combine systematic quality improvement with authentic community partnership. Successful programs recognize that evidence-based practice must include evidence from family experience (Currie et al., 2023; Gall et al., 2022; Kuo et al., 2018) and acknowledge cultural and linguistic diversity as strengths rather than barriers (Pankewicz et al., 2020). Some programs are beginning to compensate families and disabled adults for their expertise in program design, recognizing that lived experience brings valuable insight to service development (Pettigrew et al., 2024).

When service systems embrace flexible delivery models that accommodate diverse family needs, they often discover that improvements designed to benefit marginalized communities actually enhance services for everyone. For instance, offering evening appointments to accommodate working families' schedules or providing translation services not only increases access for specific populations but creates a more responsive system overall.

Conclusion

Successfully navigating services for children with developmental disabilities requires more than just understanding available resources—it demands systemic change that centers family needs and experiences at every level. This includes changes at the individual provider level, organizational or agency level, and broader policy or system-wide level. While individual families can develop strategies to coordinate care more effectively, true improvement requires transformation across these interconnected levels to create a cohesive, family-centered service environment.

Key to this transformation is acknowledging that communities—particularly families and disabled adults within them—possess crucial expertise that systems have historically overlooked. Their lived experience navigating complex systems provides essential insight for improving service delivery. When systems truly partner with families in design and evaluation, they create more effective and sustainable solutions.

The path forward requires commitment to both immediate improvements and long-term system change. This includes:

- Developing more integrated approaches to service delivery (King & Meyer, 2006)
- Creating flexible funding mechanisms that support comprehensive care (Smith & Brown, 2025)
- Building authentic partnerships with families and disabled adults (Cairncross, 2019)
- Addressing systemic inequities in service access and quality (Gall et al., 2022)

As we work toward these goals, we must remain focused on what matters most: supporting children with developmental disabilities and their families to thrive in their communities. This means moving beyond fragmented services toward truly integrated, family-centered systems of support that recognize and build upon family strengths while addressing real-world needs.

References

Adams, S., Nicholas, D., Mahant, S., Weiser, N., Kanani, R., Boydell, K., & Cohen, E. (2019). Care maps and care plans for children with medical complexity. *Child: Care, Health and Development, 45*(1), 104–110. https://doi.org/10.1111/cch.12632

Altman, L., Breen, C., Ging, J., Burrett, S., Hoffmann, T., Dickins, E., Brown, K., Zurynski, Y., & Woolfenden, S. (2018). "Dealing with the hospital has become too difficult for us to do alone"—Developing an integrated care program for children with medical complexity (CMC). *International Journal of Integrated Care, 18*(3), 14. https://doi.org/10.5334/ijic.3953

Antonelli, R. C., McAllister, J. W., & Popp, J. (2009). Making care coordination a critical component of the pediatric health system: A multidisciplinary framework. *Pediatrics, 123*(4), e978–e984. https://doi.org/10.1542/peds.2009-0915

Cairncross, N. (2019). *Family navigation as a model of care: Moving beyond the barriers* (Master's thesis, Simon Fraser University). https://summit.sfu.ca/item/18470

Children's Hospital Association. (2021). *Pediatric workforce shortages: Causes and consequences.* https://www.childrenshospitals.org

Council on Children with Disabilities and Medical Home Implementation Project Advisory Committee, Turchi, R. M., Antonelli, R. C., Norwood, K. W., Jr., Adams, R. C., Brei, T. J., Burke, R. T., Davis, B. E., Friedman, S. L., Houtrow, A. J., Kuo, D. Z., Levy, S. E., Wiley, S. E., Kalichman, M. A., Murphy, N. A., Cooley, W. C., Jeung, J., Johnson, B., Klitzner, T. S., et al. (2014). Patient- and family-centered care coordination: A framework for integrating care for children and youth across multiple systems. *Pediatrics, 133*(5), e1451–e1460. https://doi.org/10.1542/peds.2014-0318

Currie, G., Materula, D., Gall, N., Lachuk, G., Richard, C., Yohemas, M., Dewan, T., Gibbard, W. B., & Zwicker, J. (2023). Care coordination of children with neurodevelopmental disabilities and medical complexity during the COVID-19 pandemic: Caregiver experiences. *Child: Care, Health and Development, 49*(5), 834–845. https://doi.org/10.1111/cch.13149

Doucet, S., Luke, A., Splane, J., & Azar, R. (2019). Patient navigation as an approach to improve the integration of care: The case of NaviCare/SoinsNavi. *International Journal of Integrated Care, 19*(4), 7. https://doi.org/10.5334/ijic.4648

Emerson, E., & Llewellyn, G. (2021). Access to services for children with disability in rural and regional areas. *Disability & Rehabilitation, 43*(3), 342–351. https://doi.org/10.1080/09638288.2020.1731480

Family Voices. (2023). *National family survey: Children and youth with special health care needs.* https://familyvoices.org

Fong, V. C., Baumbusch, J., & Basu Khan, K. (2023). "A very different place from when the pandemic started": Lessons learned for improving systems of care for families of children with medical complexity. *Journal of Child Health Care*. Advance online publication. doi:https://doi.org/10.1177/13674935231203274

Frye, W. S., Swan, K., & Gardner, L. M. (2024). Utilization of an educational liaison for coordinated care between the medical home and school-based professionals for students with chronic pain. *Journal of School Health, 94*(3), 273–278.

Gall, V. N., Buchhalter, J., Antonelli, R. C., Richard, C., Yohemas, M., Lachuk, G., & Gibbard, W. B. (2022). Improving care for families and children with neurodevelopmental disorders and co-occurring chronic health conditions using a care coordination intervention. *Journal of Developmental & Behavioral Pediatrics, 43*(8), 444–453. https://doi.org/10.1097/DBP.0000000000001102

Houtrow, A. J., Shearer, C. S., McKernan, G., Kuhlthau, K., & Agrawal, R. (2025). Health care cost concerns and hardships for families of children with disabilities. *JAMA Network Open, 8*(4), e257826. https://doi.org/10.1001/jamanetworkopen.2025.7826

King, G., & Meyer, K. (2006). A framework of approaches for the delivery of coordinated care to children with disabilities and their families. *Journal of Disability Policy Studies, 17*(3), 156–167. https://doi.org/10.1177/10442073060170030401

Kuo, D. Z., McAllister, J. W., Rossignol, L., Turchi, R. M., & Stille, C. J. (2018). Care coordination for children with medical complexity: Whose care is it, anyway? *Pediatrics, 141*(Supplement_3), S224–S232. https://doi.org/10.1542/peds.2017-1284G

Kuo, D. Z., Houtrow, A. J., Arango, P., Kuhlthau, K. A., Simmons, J. M., & Neff, J. M. (2020). Family-centered care: Current applications and future directions in pediatric health care. *Journal of Pediatric Health Care, 34*(2), 117–127. https://doi.org/10.1016/j.pedhc.2019.10.001

Lanchak, E. R., Carter, E. W., & McMillan, E. D. (2024). "You don't know what you don't know": Parent perspectives on navigating disability-related information and resources. *Intellectual and Developmental Disabilities, 62*(6), 459–473. https://doi.org/10.1352/1934-9556-62.6.459

Luke, A., Luck, K. E., & Doucet, S. (2020). Experiences of caregivers as clients of a patient navigation program for children and youth with complex care needs: A qualitative descriptive study. *International Journal of Integrated Care, 20*(4), 10. https://doi.org/10.5334/ijic.5451

Magaña, S., Lopez, K., & Saldana, D. (2021). Barriers to autism services for Latino families: Language and trust matter. *Journal of Autism and Developmental Disorders, 51*(4), 1375–1385. https://doi.org/10.1007/s10803-020-04635-1

McAllister, J. W., McNally Keehn, R., Rodgers, R., Mpofu, P. B., Monahan, P. O., & Lock, T. M. (2018). Effects of a care coordination intervention with children with neurodevelopmental disabilities and their families. *Journal of Developmental & Behavioral Pediatrics, 39*(6). https://doi.org/10.1097/DBP.0000000000000583

Musumeci, M., & Rudowitz, R. (2022). *Medicaid services for children with special health needs: Challenges in access and support*. Kaiser Family Foundation. https://www.kff.org

Nageswaran, S., Dailey-Farley, H., & Golden, S. L. (2024). Telehealth for children with medical complexity during the COVID pandemic: A qualitative study exploring caregiver experiences. *Clinical Pediatrics, 63*(1), 53–65. https://doi.org/10.1177/00099228231204707

National Council on Disability. (2023). *Inequities in health and education services for children with disabilities*. https://ncd.gov/publications/2023

Pankewicz, A., Davis, R. K., Kim, J., Antonelli, R., Rosenberg, H., Berhane, Z., & Turchi, R. M. (2020). Children with special needs: Social determinants of health and care coordination. *Clinical Pediatrics, 59*(13), 1161–1168. https://doi.org/10.1177/0009922820941206

Parish, S. L., & Thomas, K. C. (2022). Economic disparities and family caregiving for children with disabilities. *Health Affairs, 41*(3), 417–424. https://doi.org/10.1377/hlthaff.2021.01540

Pettigrew, J., Golieb, K., & Winokur, M. (2024). Service navigation and concrete supports from a family perspective: A preventative and community-based approach to child welfare. *Children and Youth Services Review, 163*, 107793. https://doi.org/10.1016/j.childyouth.2024.107793

Sheppard, M. E., & Moran, K. K. (2022). The role of early care providers in early intervention and early childhood special education systems. *Early Childhood Education Journal, 50*(6), 891–901. https://doi.org/10.1007/s10643-021-01236-8

Smith, J. A., & Brown, L. M. (2025). Flexible grant schemes: A systematic scoping review. *Journal of Public Health Management and Practice, 31*(2), 134–142. https://doi.org/10.1097/PHH.0000000000001588

Sweet, K. S., LeBlanc, J. K., Stough, L. M., & Sweany, N. W. (2020). Community building and knowledge sharing by individuals with disabilities using social media. *Journal of Computer Assisted Learning, 36*(1), 1–11. https://doi.org/10.1111/jcal.12390

Szlamka, Z., Tekola, B., Hoekstra, R., & Hanlon, C. (2022). The role of advocacy and empowerment in shaping service development for families raising children with developmental disabilities. *Health Expectations, 25*(4), 1882–18939. https://doi.org/10.1111/hex.13539

Thibodaux, L. K., Orr, A. L., Reisinger, D. L., Fodstad, J., Xu, G., Wikel, K., & Curtin, M. (2024). A pilot study of the utility of a hospital-based school program for pediatric patients with cardiac diagnoses. *Frontiers in Pediatrics, 12*, 1502378. https://doi.org/10.3389/fped.2024.1502378

Wehmeyer, M. L., Shogren, K. A., & Kurth, J. (2021). The state of inclusion with students with intellectual and developmental disabilities in the United States. *Journal of Policy and Practice in Intellectual Disabilities, 18*(1), 36–43. https://doi.org/10.1111/jppi.12332

Whitmore, K. E., Johnson, N. L., Park, S., Salama, S., & Sobiesk, R. J. (2023). Improving inclusion for children with special health care needs in childcare settings: Results from a statewide survey of childcare professionals. *Journal of Pediatric Health Care, 37*(2), e1–e10. https://doi.org/10.1016/j.pedhc.2022.10.011

Zuckerman, K. E., Sinche, B., Cobian, M., Cervantes, M., Mejia, A., & Nicolaidis, C. (2021). Racial disparities in early childhood service access among children with developmental delays. *Pediatrics, 147*(6), e2020010100. https://doi.org/10.1542/peds.2020-010100

Chapter 11
Systems of Care and Policy to Improve Resilience of Young Children with Developmental Disabilities and Health Conditions

Jennifer Marshall, Joanna F. Mackie, Acadia W. Buro, Rafaella Stein Elger, Suman Kanti Chowdhury, and Russell S. Kirby

Abstract This chapter examines the development and current state of systems of care and policy frameworks designed to strengthen resilience in young children with developmental disabilities and health conditions, known as children with special healthcare needs (CSHCN). Using both person-centered and identity-first language, it stresses the vital need for integrated medical, behavioral, educational, and social services that provide comprehensive support. Synthesizing key models—such as the Social Ecological Model, Life Course Theory, and Resilience Theory—it illustrates how child well-being results from dynamic interactions among individual traits, family dynamics, community resources, and broader policy and cultural factors. The chapter reviews prevalence statistics, disparities in access, and the evolution of support systems, noting how structural inequities hinder equitable outcomes. It highlights the collective responsibility of communities, families, and institutions to build adaptive, inclusive systems that foster participation, well-being, and rights for all children, concluding with a call for integrated, equitable care aligned across policy, practice, and research to support children and families.

Keywords Children with special healthcare needs · Systems of care · Collaborative efforts · Community-based supports · Social ecological model · Medical home · Adverse childhood experiences · Policy

J. Marshall (✉) · R. S. Elger · S. K. Chowdhury · R. S. Kirby
College of Public Health, University of South Florida, Tampa, FL, USA
e-mail: jm@usf.edu

J. F. Mackie
Department of Population Health Sciences, University of Central Florida, Orlando, FL, USA

A. W. Buro
College of Population Health, University of New Mexico Health Sciences Center, Albuquerque, NM, USA

L. Nabors and T. Stanton-Chapman (eds.), *Developmental Disabilities and Chronic Illness in Young Children*, Springer Series on Child and Family Studies,
https://doi.org/10.1007/978-3-032-08523-8_11

Children make up 20–25% of the population, yet stand apart from adults in our consideration of their personhood and need for protections. The role of a child's primary parent or caregiver has always been and continues to be paramount. However, the adage "it takes a village to raise a child" remains equally true. Our community, national and global villages have grappled with the extent to which society and communities play a role in directly supporting children's health and development. The United Nations Convention on the Rights of the Child (UNRCRC, 1989) and the United Nations Convention and the Rights of Persons with Disabilities (CRPD, 2006) call for recognition of the human rights to participate fully in all aspects of society, to be protected from any form of discrimination, and to be provided every opportunity to thrive regardless of context. Throughout history, other global and United States' (U.S.) national conventions, policy statements, national organizations, and legislation around the health, education, care, and protection of children have arisen.

Our society has not always played a role in protecting or promoting the health, safety, and well-being of children (Dawes, et al., 2022). Historically this responsibility has fallen under the purview of parents/caregivers rather than the collective. From the late nineteenth to mid-twentieth centuries, key historical events precipitated the emergence of public systems to support children's health and wellness, especially in the context of two major time periods: the Great Depression in the 1930s and the Great Society in the 1960s and 1970s. While the field of pediatrics as a specialty began in 1888 it was not until 1930 that the American Academy of Pediatrics was founded (Mahnke, 2000). Around the same time, in 1933, early—albeit temporary—federal support for out-of-home child care became available in the form of Emergency Nursery Schools as part of the Works Progress Administration, primarily to help families struggling with intense poverty (Cohen, 1996). Another temporary effort occurred during World War II, when there was federal investment in public child care via the Lanham Act of 1941. Public investment in child care did not become permanent until Head Start was launched in 1965, and continues to this day (Cohen, 1996). Similarly, the 1938 Fair Labor Act, which set a minimum wage and minimum age of 16 for work in mining or manufacturing, was in response to large numbers of children, including small children, working in dangerous conditions due to unprecedented numbers of families suffering in extreme poverty. (Forsythe, 1939).

The modern concept of child welfare and child protection as a public responsibility began in 1962 with the publication of a paper by a physician, Henry Kempe, titled "Battered Child Syndrome," which articulated a problem that had been previously observed but not recognized as requiring intervention outside the family (Kempe et al., 1962). Experts in child health also began to set guidelines and expectations for the specific health needs of children, such as newborn screening (El-Hattab et al., 2018), and developmental screening requirements through EPSDT (Peters, 2006) and CAPTA (Stoltzfus, E. (2009). The National School Lunch Act was established in 1946, expanded in 1968 to include breakfast (Ralston et al., 2008), and in 1972 the supplemental nutrition program for Women, Infants and Children (WIC) began providing services to eligible women and children (U.S. Department of Agriculture, 2024). The field of Infant Mental Health (IMH) also emerged in the 1970s, when developmental psychologists became interested in the significance of early childhood experiences. Attachment theory proposed that healthy social and emotional development depended on healthy relationships with others, beginning, for infants, with their primary caregiver (Simpson et al., 2016). The dyadic focus of IMH reinforces the critical role of parents and caregivers for young children's healthy development. Historically many public systems and supports for children emerged in response to specific events or circumstances, and currently there is a need for sustained and coordinated federal investments in young children and their families (Halfon et al., 2024).

Similarly, protections and considerations for people with disabilities slowly evolved over time. While "people with disabilities" is widely used in health and policy fields, many individuals prefer "disabled people" to affirm disability as a valued part of their identity, this work respects and reflects both perspectives. The Americans with Disabilities Act (ADA) (1990) prohibits discrimination against people with disabilities in all settings. The foundational Education for All Handicapped Children Act (Education for All Handicapped Children Act of 1975, 1975) of 1975, later referred to as the Individuals with Disabilities Education Act and reauthorized in 2004 (IDEA, 2004) states that every child, including those with disabilities, had the right to a "free, appropriate, public education" and framed public education as a right rather than a privilege.

This chapter provides an overview of the relevant theories that underpin policies, programs, and overarching systems of care for children in the United States, specifically children with special healthcare needs. There is still more to be done, with particular challenges in the implementation of these policies and adherence. Some of those challenges and goals for the future will be described in the discussion.

Children with Special Healthcare Needs

Every year, nearly 3.7 million babies are born in the United States (Osterman et al., 2021). Defining and characterizing the population of infants and children with complex and chronic medical conditions has evolved over the past century from 'crippled children's programs' in the 1930s through a more generic noncategorical term of 'children with chronic health needs' in 1981 (Perrin et al., 1993). Today, they are commonly known as children with special healthcare needs (CSHCN), a term adopted in 1998 by the Maternal and Child Health Bureau (MCHB) under the Health Resources and Services Administration (HRSA). The MCHB defines CSHCN as *"those who have or are at increased risk for a chronic physical, developmental, behavioral, or emotional condition and who also require health and related services of a type or amount beyond that required by children generally"* (McPherson et al., 1998). The acronym CYSHCN (children and youth with special healthcare needs) includes individuals up to age 21. CSHCN form a diverse group of children who require health and related services beyond those typically required by their peers. The term was established by the MCHB to capture the broad spectrum of children with medical or support needs stemming from complex health conditions, ranging from chronic illnesses such as asthma and diabetes to developmental disabilities like autism and Down syndrome. As language evolved to align with more inclusive, empowering, and strengths-based perspectives, alternatives to "CSHCN" such as "children requiring additional support," "children with disabilities," "children with complex needs," and other terms have been used to describe a subset or all of CHSCN (Gernsbacher et al., 2016). It is also important to note that while people-first language has been encouraged to emphasize the individual before their diagnosis, more recently many within the disability community, particularly those who embrace disability pride, prefer identity-first language (e.g., "autistic person"), seeing their disability as an integral and valued part of who they are. Recognizing and respecting individual preferences in language is essential in fostering a more person-centered and affirming approach to discussing disability and support needs (Grech et al., 2023). We use the term CSHCN for consistency with federal definitions and surveillance data, while acknowledging its limitations and the importance of language that reflects evolving perspectives and lived experiences.

To determine whether a child has special healthcare needs, the MCHB's need-based definition includes five consequences—(1) need for prescription medicine, (2) beyond average need or use of medical, mental health or educational services, (3) functional limitations compared with others of same age, (4) need of specialized therapies, and (5) treatment or counseling for emotional or developmental problems (Ghandour et al., 2022). If one or more of these consequences arise from medical or other health conditions and persist for 12 months or longer, the child is classified as having special healthcare needs (Child & Adolescent Health Measurement Initiative, n.d.).

Within the population of CSHCN are infants born with congenital conditions. The National Birth Defects Prevention Network (NBDPN https://nbdpn.org/) currently consists of 40 state birth defects surveillance programs that collaborate on creating technical guidelines for conducting epidemiological surveillance of children born with a defined set of 45 congenital and metabolic conditions. Data on maternal and infant characteristics (maternal race, ethnicity, age at delivery, year of delivery and infant sex) as well as pregnancy outcomes for these cases are also collected. Birth defects surveillance helps to better understand the prevalence rates, trends, risk factors, and outcomes for these children. Since 1997, the NBDPN has created annual reports and data tables, and currently facilitates collaborative efforts to disseminate findings overall and for specific conditions or affected sub-populations.

Infants may also develop medical and health complexities or developmental disabilities after birth or throughout their childhood; estimating their prevalence and outcomes is more challenging. Currently, approximately one in five children under 18 years in the United States or about 14 million children have special healthcare needs (Ghandour et al., 2022). The prevalence varies geographically, ranging from 14% in Hawaii to 24% in West Virginia. The burden of special needs is disproportionately higher among older boys from economically disadvantaged families compared to children generally (Houtrow et al., 2022). According to the 2022–2023 National Survey of Children's Health, 20.8% (95% CI 20.4–21.3) of children in the United

States qualify as CSHCN (CAHMI, retrieved June 21, 2025). However, significant disparities exist in the prevalence, outcomes, and access to care for CYSHCN, disproportionately affecting children from racial and ethnic minority groups, low-income families, and rural communities. Structural inequities, systemic racism, and under-resourced healthcare and educational systems exacerbate these disparities, creating barriers to achieving health equity for CSHCN (Houtrow et al., 2022). Some multi-state networks focus on specific developmental disabilities, such as the Autism and Developmental Disabilities Monitoring Network which tracks autism and cerebral palsy in specific locales (CDC, n.d.). While some states have databases that include children participating in programs, such as early intervention or special education programs (e.g., California Department of Developmental Services), truly population-based longitudinal data on healthcare utilization and developmental outcomes for children with special needs are largely unavailable. Population-based data concerning the prevalence of CSHCN were historically difficult to obtain prior to the creation of the National Survey of Children's Health (NSCH) and the companion National Survey of Children with Special Healthcare Needs. These surveys, funded by the federal Maternal and Child Health Bureau and managed by the National Center for Health Statistics and the US Bureau of the Census, provide national and state-level data on the prevalence of specific health conditions affecting children 0–17 years of age, as well as factors influencing their health status and access to care (Ghandour et al., 2018). Research on access to a medical home and outcomes on a population basis are generally unavailable, but inferences can be made from the NSCH as well as smaller clinical research studies. Research on outcomes associated with systems of care for CSHCN is also limited.

Over the past decades, overall life expectancy of CSHCN has improved due to advancements in medical care, advent of technologies, societal inclusion, and policy support (Irving et al., 2008). Currently, more than 90% of CSHCN in the U.S. survive through adulthood with about half a million turn to 18 years each year (Nugent et al., 2018). However, compared to children in general, CSHCN have high unmet needs (Huang et al., 2020) and less than half of these children receive care within a medical home (Coller et al., 2020; Ghandour et al., 2022; Lichstein et al., 2018). Outcomes for CSHCN vary widely depending on individual, family, and systemic factors. Addressing inequities requires a shift toward health equity-focused models of care that prioritize reducing barriers for CSHCN and their families. This involves promoting policies and systems that ensure equitable access to healthcare, inclusive educational environments, and community supports. For example, family-centered care models and community-based supports tailored to specific cultural and linguistic needs can significantly improve outcomes (Houtrow et al., 2022). Additionally, greater integration of health, education, and social service systems is needed to address the systemic barriers that disproportionately impact certain demographic groups of CSHCN.

Systems

A systems perspective is critical for understanding the complexity of children's development and involves a holistic view. Systems-informed theories of child development typically involve interconnected and interdependent elements of influence, such as a child, their family and home environment, their school, community, and broader society (Masten, 2018). Further, a change in one aspect of a system may ripple through the entire network. Systems involve dynamic interactions and feedback loops, with some elements directly influencing the child (e.g., their parents) while other elements influence the child in a much more indirect way (e.g., their parents' paid leave policies).

The systems perspective is particularly appropriate in the context of children's health and development (Guralnick, 2011), as growth and development are dynamic, constantly changing with time and the influences of various aspects of their environments. A systems perspective provides context for interventions that may only focus on one aspect of the system (e.g., healthcare/pediatrician, education/IEP, family services) viewed individually may tell a different story compared with viewing the whole child across their system of care. *A classic example is a child who seems to be acting out and identified for a behavioral consultation in preschool, only to be assessed and realize it is the child's hearing that is the problem. Viewing their behavior alone does not tell the whole story.*

The Developmental Systems Approach combines several disciplines, including biology and psychology, to illustrate the temporal dynamic nature and evolution in human development. This approach emphasizes the core principles of relationships, comprehensiveness, and continuity of child and family support to optimize development (Guralnick, 2020). The Developmental Systems approach explains how children's inherent developmental resources and processes are influenced by family interactions, which are drawn from caregiver characteristics and resources. The caregiver-child dyad is central in many developmental theories and models, and plays a central role in shaping a child's well-being (Ornstein & Caruso, 2024). More broadly, the Ecological Systems Theory of Child Development posits that children's health and well-being is influenced by various systems across their lives, including formal systems such as health, safety, and education, and informal systems such as families, communities, and society (Olson, 1965; Ostrom, 1990).

Conceptual Frameworks

Conceptual frameworks serve as critical tools for understanding the experiences of CSHCN and guiding research, practice, and policy development. These frameworks provide a structured way to understand interactions between individual needs, environmental supports, and systemic barriers.

Family Systems Theory views the family as an interconnected emotional unit, emphasizing the dynamic relationships between members rather than focusing on individuals in isolation (Bowen, 1966; Calatrava et al., 2022). Originally developed in clinical psychology, this framework highlights how emotions and behaviors are transmitted across generations, shaping family dynamics over time. Applied to CSHCN, the theory underscores the importance of integrated care systems that support both the child and their family as a whole (Kuo et al., 2022). Research exploring family perspectives on Down syndrome aligns with these principles, demonstrating how emotions, attitudes, and coping mechanisms are shared among parents, siblings, and the individual with Down syndrome (Skotko et al., 2016). These studies show that having a child with Down syndrome influences family roles, stress levels, and adaptation processes, reinforcing the theory's emphasis on interconnectedness and collective adjustment (Hodapp, 2007). The theory also provides insight into how family support systems impact a child's development, as children who feel supported are more likely to develop a strong self-concept and thrive in social and academic settings. By recognizing families as interdependent systems, Family Systems Theory offers a valuable framework for identifying unmet support needs, including care coordination and mental health services, ensuring a holistic approach to the well-being of CSHCN and their families.

Bronfenbrenner's **Social Ecological Model** illustrates how a child's development is shaped by multiple overlapping systems, ranging from immediate family, community, and school environments to broader societal influences (Bronfenbrenner, 1977, 1979). At the microsystem level, direct interactions with family, healthcare providers, and caregivers play a crucial role. For example, mothers of CSHCN often serve as primary caregivers while facing social isolation and the need for community support (Kikuhara et al., 2021). The mesosystem represents the connections between different environments in a child's life, such as the interaction between home, healthcare, and education systems. An example of this is the collaboration between healthcare providers and educational institutions to support CSHCN's development and well-being (Warren et al., 2022). The exosystem consists of external influences that indirectly impact children, such as community resources, social networks, and healthcare infrastructure. For instance, social capital and community-based services play a significant role in determining the accessibility of healthcare for CSHCN (Pennington et al., 2021). The macrosystem encompasses broader societal and cultural influences, including policies and systemic factors that shape healthcare and social services. Addressing racial disparities and promoting health equity, for example, are essential for improving outcomes for CSHCN (Dawson et al., 2022). Finally, the chronosystem refers to changes over time that influence a child's development, such as shifts in healthcare policies that affect service availability. The model also acknowledges individual-level factors, including biological and genetic characteristics, which interact with these broader systems. For example, children with chronic kidney disease (CKD) may experience stress differently due to their condition, necessitating personalized care approaches (Dawson et al., 2022). By emphasizing these interconnected layers, the Social Ecological Model provides a comprehensive framework for understanding the diverse factors that shape the health and well-being of CSHCN and highlights its relevance in addressing systemic disparities in healthcare.

The **Life Course Theory** provides a framework for understanding how health and developmental outcomes are shaped by experiences across the lifespan. Historically, MCH research has focused on contemporaneous risk factors, but increasing MCH concerns in the U.S. over the past three decades have shifted attention toward the long-term health impacts of exposures, behaviors, and experiences, including intergenerational influences (Kotch, 2013). The concept gained notoriety in 1997 with the introduction of life course epidemiology (Kuh & Ben-Shlomo, 1997), followed by influential work on racial disparities in birth outcomes (Lu & Halfon, 2003) and MCHB's 75th anniversary report, which reinforced the importance of a life course approach in MCH policy (United States Maternal and Child Health Bureau, 2010). Life Course Theory serves as both a theoretical framework for guiding research and a conceptual tool for understanding sequences of life events. As a theory, it emphasizes that health is shaped by lifelong processes, individual choices, the timing of experiences, social relationships, and historical context (Elder, 2006). It also introduces three key concepts: trajectories, which describe patterns of health across time; turning points, which mark significant shifts in life direction; and transitions, which are short-term changes embedded within trajectories. The theory has been widely applied in fields such as life course epidemiology, preconception health, adverse childhood experiences, and fetal origins of adult diseases; for example, the importance of folic acid supplementation before pregnancy in preventing neural tube defects illustrates how early-life interventions can influence long-term health trajectories. Its policy and practice implications highlight the need for integrated, comprehensive services that recognize the cumulative nature of health and emphasize continuity of care across life stages.

The **Adverse Childhood Experiences** conceptual model examines the impact of adverse childhood experiences (ACEs) on health outcomes. ACEs are potentially traumatic events occurring before age 18 that can have long-term consequences for health and well-being (Boullier & Blair, 2018). These include experiences of violence, abuse, neglect, exposure to household mental health or substance use issues, and witnessing violence. ACEs are linked to increased risks of mental health disorders, risky behaviors, substance use, chronic disease, toxic stress, and premature death (Crouch et al., 2019). Among CSHCN, 53% have experienced at least one ACE, a significantly higher prevalence compared to the general population (Stein Elger et al., 2023). Exposure to ACEs also increases the likelihood of having special healthcare needs, with family and community-level ACEs particularly associated with CSHCN status (Kan et al., 2020). Addressing ACEs within systems of care requires provider training, routine screening, and integration into prevention and early childhood programs such as home visiting (McKelvey et al., 2016). Additionally, achieving health equity for CSHCN requires addressing the broader social determinants that contribute to ACEs, such as poverty and discrimination, through cross-sector collaboration, policy reform, and community engagement (Houtrow et al., 2022).

Conversely, **Positive Childhood Experiences** (PCEs) serve as protective factors that promote resilience and well-being. While the concept is more recent, it emphasizes the role of interpersonal and community supports in mitigating the impact of ACEs (Huang et al., 2023). PCEs, such as participating in after-school activities, having a guiding mentor, and living in a supportive neighborhood, are associated with lower risks of poor physical and mental health outcomes in adulthood (Baglivio & Wolff, 2020; Crouch et al., 2023). Recognizing the dual importance of reducing ACEs and fostering PCEs within systems of care is essential to improving long-term outcomes for CSHCN.

According to the **Resilience Theory**, protective factors such as strong relationships, access to supportive services, and adaptive coping strategies play a critical role in fostering resilience in the face of adversity (Masten & Cicchetti, 2016). For example, children who feel supported by their families and communities are more likely to develop a positive self-concept and flourish in social and academic settings. The context in which these protective factors operate is equally essential. The broader environment in which these protective factors operate is equally significant, as inclusive spaces—such as playgrounds designed for all children—can facilitate meaningful interactions and positive developmental outcomes.

The **Medical Home** model, recommended by the American Academy of Pediatrics, is particularly important for CSHCN, including those with autism (Hyman et al., 2020; Rast et al., 2021; Shi et al., 2017). This patient-centered approach provides comprehensive and cost-effective care through an integrated, multidisciplinary team that ensures both primary and specialty care are coordinated and cohesive (Mendel et al., 2018; Rast et al., 2021). Care delivered within this model is expected to be compassionate, family-centered, continuous, comprehensive, coordinated, culturally responsive, and accessible (Carbone et al., 2010; Dang et al., 2017; Hyman et al., 2020; Rast et al., 2021). Functioning as a partnership between healthcare providers, patients, and families, the medical home seeks to optimize health outcomes and overall care quality (Cene et al., 2016; Cheak-Zamora & Farmer, 2015). Access to a medical home is typically assessed based on five key components: having a usual source of care, a personal doctor or nurse, family-centered care, the ability to obtain referrals, and access to care coordination services (Cheak-Zamora & Farmer, 2015; Kogan et al., 2008; Rast et al., 2021). For children with autism, this model is particularly beneficial due to their complex healthcare needs and co-occurring conditions, as it facilitates access to developmental resources, screenings, and ongoing surveillance (Cheak-Zamora & Farmer, 2015; Ming et al., 2011; Rast et al., 2021). More broadly, the medical home framework prioritizes preventive and proactive management of health concerns, reducing reliance on crisis-driven interventions for CSHCN (Aguayo et al., 2024). Additionally, it plays a crucial role in addressing racial and ethnic disparities in mental health access, as these gaps often result from differences in practice behaviors and preexisting barriers to care (Rast et al., 2024). By emphasizing continuity, coordination, and accessibility, the medical home model offers a structured approach to improving long-term health outcomes for CSHCN.

Family-Centered Care (FCC) is a healthcare approach that emphasizes collaboration between healthcare providers, patients, and families to ensure care is respectful, inclusive, and responsive to individual needs (Johnson et al., 2008). As a core component of the medical home model, FCC recognizes families as integral members of the care team, particularly in decision-making for CSHCN (Bellizzi et al., 2021). The framework is built on four key principles: dignity and respect, information sharing, participation, and collaboration (Hsu et al., 2019). By honoring the strengths, cultures, and expertise of both families and professionals, FCC fosters partnerships that improve health outcomes and enhance the well-being of children and their families (Arango, 2011; Family Voices, 2025). Despite its benefits, disparities in FCC persist. Families of children with autism and developmental delays report lower satisfaction with care due to providers' limited understanding, rigid protocols, and a lack of accommodations (Kindratt et al., 2022; Kouo et al., 2022). Black and Hispanic children, as well as those from low-income or non-English-speaking households, are less likely to receive culturally competent care or sufficient provider engagement (Morgan et al., 2022). By addressing these disparities and ensuring FCC principles are fully integrated into systems of care, healthcare providers can better support the diverse and complex needs of CSHCN and their families.

Parents want and need community supports incorporated into healthcare (Son et al., 2018). The systems of care framework provides a coordinated, community-based approach to delivering services for children with special healthcare needs (CSHCN), emphasizing integration, collaboration, and accessibility (Stroul & Friedman, 1986). Initially developed to address gaps in mental health services, the framework has evolved to support a broader population, including children at risk for developmental, behavioral, and medical challenges (Stroul et al., 2010). Rather than a rigid model, systems of care serve as a guiding philosophy that adapts to the needs of the child, family, and community. Its core principles prioritize reducing reliance on restrictive care settings, enhancing family and youth partnerships, and ensuring culturally and linguistically appropriate services (Stroul et al., 2010; Stroul & Blau, 2010). Research has shown that adherence to this framework leads to improved family and child outcomes, better coordination among service providers, and a shift toward preventive, community-based care (Stroul et al., 2012; Williams et al., 2021).

For CSHCN, implementing systems of care involves integrating medical, behavioral, educational, and social services to create a seamless continuum of care. These systems encompass diagnosis, screening, referrals, early intervention, behavioral and therapeutic support, skill development, and care coordination (Lubetsky et al., 2014). While medical homes share similar principles, they primarily focus on healthcare, whereas systems of care extend across multiple service domains (Mendel et al., 2018; Rast et al., 2021). Successful implementation has led to policy changes, increased provider training, expanded community-based mental health services, and strengthened partnerships between families, providers, and community organizations (Lubetsky et al., 2014). However, gaps remain, particularly in ensuring equitable access to services, training providers in interdisciplinary care, and expanding behavioral health supports (Lubetsky et al., 2014). By fostering integration across service systems, the framework enhances care accessibility, improves outcomes, and strengthens long-term support for CSHCN and their families.

Policy Driven Systems of Care Informed by History, Theory, and Society

Health

Promoting health services in a well-functioning system has been a central focus and national priority in the United States for CSHCN due to the presence of chronic illnesses or developmental disabilities. System of care is an approach to provide a comprehensive network of services and support for these children in a coordinated, family-oriented way, and easily accessible health services across the lifespan (Association of Maternal and Child Health Programs, 2017). The MCHB identifies a well-functioning system of care if it—(1) includes families as a partner in decision-making, (2) provides early and regular screening services, (3) makes services organized for easy access, (4) allows children receiving services in a medical home, (5) offers adequate health insurance, and (6) provides transition support to adult care.

Receiving care within a medical home has consistently been shown to benefit CSHCN. Medical home is a well-recognized approach in primary care that provides comprehensive health services in an organized, family-centered, uninterrupted, empathetic, and culturally appropriate manner (American Academy of Pediatrics (AAP), 2002). Children who receive care within a medical home tend to experience less delayed care, fewer unmet healthcare needs, higher preventive medical visits, and fewer emergency visits (Strickland et al., 2009; Willits et al., 2013). Family-centered care and care coordination also have shown positive influences on health outcomes for young children with chronic illness or developmental disabilities. When health services are provided in an environment where family members are actively involved in the planning and decision-making process, the child's developmental outcomes tend to be more favorable, and the patient (e.g., parent, child) is more satisfied with the health services (Mestre et al., 2024).

Examples of Systems

Head Start is a federal-to-local program that started in 1965 as part of the War of Poverty policy initiative. It began as an 8-week summer program that quickly grew into a system serving more than 800,000 children annually, including almost 250,000 infants and toddlers in Early Head Start, 245,000 preschoolers, more than 20,000 Alaska Native American Indian children, and more than 20,000 children in Migrant Head Start. Head Start also serves more than 12,000 pregnant women through Early

Head Start annually. In addition to early childhood education, Head Start includes many whole child/whole family services, such as health, development, hearing, and vision screenings; meals and nutrition counseling; prenatal services for pregnant women; job training and adult education; home visiting and parent engagement; and connecting families with a medical home (US DHHS, n.d.). Recognizing the positive effects of early education for young children with disabilities, in 1972 Congress mandated that Head Start programs enroll at least 10% children with disabilities (Lee & Luellen, 2021). Today Head Start implements practices from the Universal Design for Learning (UDL), which involves proactively structing the environment and practices to include all children by allowing for multiple means of engagement, expression, and representation (Lohnmann et al., 2018). Evidence indicates that Head Start is effective for children with disabilities who attend. One study found that among children with disabilities, those enrolled in Head Start for at least 1 year had better cognitive outcomes at age 4 and age 6 compared with similar children not enrolled in Head Start (Lee & Luellen, 2021). Other studies show the benefit of inclusion for all children, including children without special healthcare needs (Kart & Kart, 2021).

Home visiting programs are a system of family supports that use a community-based approach, with more than 3000 programs operating across the United States, typically serving young children or those with significant medical needs (Johnson, 2011). These programs are built on evidence-based models that emphasize the importance of early childhood development, demonstrating positive outcomes in children's health and family well-being (Kotch, 2013). By engaging with families in their home environments, providers can tailor services to meet each child's specific needs. The Maternal, Infant, and Early Childhood Home Visiting program supports these initiatives at the state level, ensuring that federally funded programs adhere to rigorous evidence-based standards (Health Resources & Services Administration, n.d.). Another key example is the home-based option of Early Head Start (EHS), which provides families with individualized support focused on child development, health, and school readiness. EHS home-based programs traditionally offer weekly 90-min in-person home visits that are structured to promote parent-child interactions and reinforce early learning (Vicente et al., 2022). As a two-generation program, EHS also aims to enhance family self-sufficiency, with research demonstrating its long-term benefits, including improvements in children's social-emotional development and increased family income 2 years after program completion (Jones Harden et al., 2012).

Recreational and inclusive community programs offer children with disabilities opportunities for physical and social engagement. Special Olympics is a prominent example, providing year-round training and competition in 33 Olympic-style sports for children and adults with intellectual disabilities (Myśliwiec & Damentko, 2015). Participation in Special Olympics has been shown to improve physical health, enhance social skills, and build self-confidence in a supportive and inclusive environment (Turgeon et al., 2023). The program also plays a broader role in promoting societal inclusion by challenging stereotypes and engaging over five million athletes worldwide (McConkey et al., 2022). These types of programs help children with special healthcare needs develop critical life skills while fostering a sense of belonging within their communities.

Parent education, support, and family-centered care interventions further expand support systems for families of children with disabilities (Vanegas & Abdelrahim, 2016). For example, intensive caregiver education programs have been widely implemented to equip parents with the necessary knowledge and skills to manage their child's health needs effectively, leading to improved caregiver self-sufficiency and enhanced access to community resources. Support groups offer additional benefits by providing caregivers with spaces to share experiences and receive emotional support, ultimately improving outcomes for both children and families (Watkinson et al., 2023). Technological innovations such as mobile health tracking interventions have also been developed to enhance family-centered care, allowing caregivers to monitor their child's health metrics while improving communication with healthcare providers (Watkinson et al., 2023). Similarly, family empowerment programs focus on strengthening caregivers' knowledge and advocacy skills, leading to increased access to necessary services and improved long-term outcomes for children (Casagrande & Ingersoll, 2021).

By integrating home visiting programs, inclusive recreational opportunities, parent-mediated interventions, and caregiver support initiatives, community-based interventions serve as a critical component of the broader system of care for CSHCN. These programs bridge gaps between health, education, and social services, ensuring that children and their families receive the resources and support needed to thrive. Their emphasis on accessibility, empowerment, and continuity of care contributes to improved developmental outcomes and long-term family well-being, reinforcing the importance of community-driven approaches in supporting CSHCN.

Conclusion

The way society conceptualizes disability has evolved over time, moving from a medical model that focuses on deficits to a social model that recognizes social and environmental barriers (Oliver, 1990, 2013). This shift reframes the conversation around disability from one limitation to one of inclusion, empowerment, and quality of life (Lollar & Crews, 2003). The Social Model of Disability challenges traditional medical perspectives by framing disability not as an individual deficit but as the result of social, political, and environmental barriers, affirming that disability arises from societal barriers rather than individual impairments (Constantino et al., 2022; McDonald & Raymaker, 2013; Oliver, 2013). Critical Disability Theory, increasingly recognizes the role of systemic inequities in shaping the experiences of children with disabilities, highlighting the need for policies and practices that promote equity and participation to combat ableism (the belief that being non-disabled is the norm) and systemic exclusion (Rocco, 2005; Procknow et al., 2017) by recognizing that disability exists within a continuum, shaped by lived experiences and broader social power relations, while also emphasizing intersectionality and the influence of race, gender, class, and sexuality in shaping disabled identities (Reaume, 2014). By reframing disability as a product of exclusion rather than impairment, Critical Disability Theory promotes accessible, inclusive environments that center the voices and expertise of disabled individuals (Hall, 2019).

Because the future policy landscape is uncertain, and federal supports may be reduced, state and local communities may need to re-envision systems of care and support toward a more universal model. Overall, to ensure the well—being of CSHCN, our society must continue to embrace the conceptual shift that recognizes the importance of systems of care that support children and their families (United Nations, 1989) while also recognizing the right to inclusion, participation, self-determination, and dignity for individuals with disabilities as fundamental human rights (Berghs et al., 2019; Bollinger & Cook, 2020; Reaume, 2014; Russo & Wooley, 2020).

References

Aguayo, P., Lin, A. G., Stevens, P. T., Carbone, P. S., Bilder, D. A., & Rapaport, M. H. (2024). A patient-centered multidisciplinary medical HOME for persons with intellectual and developmental disabilities. *Focus, 22*(2), 170–174. https://doi.org/10.1176/appi.focus.20230036

American Academy of Pediatrics. (2002). The medical home. *Pediatrics, 110*(1), 184–186. https://doi.org/10.1542/peds.110.1.184

Americans With Disabilities Act of 1990, 42 U.S.C. § 12101 et seq. (1990). https://www.ada.gov/pubs/adastatute08.htm

Arango, P. (2011). Family-centered care. *Academic Pediatrics, 11*(2), 97–99. https://doi.org/10.1016/j.acap.2010.12.004

Association of Maternal and Child Health Programs. (2017). *Standards for systems of care for children and youth with special health care needs version* 2.0. https://amchp.org/resources/standards-for-systems-of-care-for-children-and-youth-with-special-health-care-needs-version-2-0/

Baglivio, M. T., & Wolff, K. T. (2020). Positive childhood experiences (PCE): Cumulative resiliency in the face of adverse childhood experiences. *Youth Violence and Juvenile Justice, 19*(2), 139–162. https://doi.org/10.1177/1541204020972487

Bellizzi, S., Pichierri, G., & Panu Napodano, C. M. (2021). Family-centered care for children during pandemics. *Public Health, 198*, e9–e10. https://doi.org/10.1016/j.puhe.2021.04.016

Berghs, M., Atkin, K., Hatton, C., & Thomas, C. (2019). Do disabled people need a stronger social model: A social model of human rights? *Disability & Society, 34*(7–8), 1034–1039. https://doi.org/10.1080/09687599.2019.1619239

Bollinger, H., & Cook, H. (2020). After the social model: Young physically disabled people, sexuality education and sexual experience. *Journal of Youth Studies, 23*(7), 837–852. https://doi.org/10.1080/13676261.2019.1639647

Boullier, M., & Blair, M. (2018). Adverse childhood experiences. *Paediatrics and Child Health, 28*(3), 132–137. https://doi.org/10.1016/j.paed.2017.12.008

Bowen, M. (1966). The use of family theory in clinical practice. *Comprehensive Psychiatry, 7*(5), 345–374. https://doi.org/10.1016/S0010-440X(66)80065-2

Bronfenbrenner, U. (1977). Toward an experimental ecology of human development. *American Psychologist, 32*(7), 513–531. https://doi.org/10.1037/0003-066X.32.7.513

Bronfenbrenner, U. (1979). *The ecology of human development: Experiments by nature and design.* Harvard University Press.

Calatrava, M., Martins, M. V., Schweer-Collins, M., Duch-Ceballos, C., & Rodríguez-González, M. (2022). Differentiation of self: A scoping review of Bowen family systems theory's core construct. *Clinical Psychology Review, 91*, 102101. https://doi.org/10.1016/j.cpr.2021.102101
Carbone, P. S., Behl, D. D., Azor, V., & Murphy, N. A. (2010). The medical home for children with autism spectrum disorders: Parent and pediatrician perspectives. *Journal of Autism and Developmental Disorders, 40*(3), 317–324. https://doi.org/10.1007/s10803-009-0874-5
Casagrande, K., & Ingersoll, B. R. (2021). Improving service access in ASD: A aystematic review of family empowerment interventions for children with special healthcare needs. *Journal of Autism and Developmental Disorders, 8*(2), 170–185. https://doi.org/10.1007/s40489-020-002 08-9
Cene, C. W., Johnson, B. H., Wells, N., Baker, B., Davis, R., & Turchi, R. (2016). A narrative review of patient and family engagement: The "Foundation" of the Medical "Home". *Medical Care, 54*(7), 697–705. https://doi.org/10.1097/MLR.0000000000000548
Centers for Disease Control and Prevention (CDC). (n.d.). *Autism and Developmental Disabilities Monitoring (ADDM) Network*. Autism Spectrum Disorder (ASD). https://www.cdc.gov/autism/addm-network/index.html
Cheak-Zamora, N. C., & Farmer, J. E. (2015). The impact of the medical home on access to care for children with autism spectrum disorders. *Journal of Autism and Developmental Disorders, 45*(3), 636–644. https://doi.org/10.1007/s10803-014-2218-3
Child & Adolescent Health Measurement Initiative. 2022–2023 National Survey of Children's Health (NSCH) data query. Data Resource Center for Child and Adolescent Health supported by the U.S. Department of Health and Human Services, Health Resources and Services Administration (HRSA), Maternal and Child Health Bureau (MCHB). Retrieved January 28, 2025 from www.childhealthdata.org
Child & Adolescent Health Measurement Initiative. (n.d.). Resources. *Children With Special Health Care Needs (CSHCN) Screener.* Retrieved June 21, 2025 from https://www.cahmi.org/resources
Cohen, A. J. (1996). A brief history of federal support for child care in the United States. *The Future of Children, 6*(2), 26–40. https://doi.org/10.2307/1602417
Coller, R. J., Ahrens, S., Ehlenbach, M. L., Shadman, K. A., Mathur, M., Caldera, K., Chung, P. J., LaRocque, A., Peto, H., Binger, K., Smith, W., & Sheehy, A. (2020). Priorities and outcomes for youth-adult transitions in hospital care: Perspectives of inpatient clinical leaders at US children's hospitals. *Hospital Pediatrics, 10*(9), 774–782. https://doi.org/10.1542/hpeds.2020-0016
Constantino, C., Campbell, P., & Simpson, S. (2022). Stuttering and the social model. *Journal of Communication Disorders, 96*, 106200. https://doi.org/10.1016/j.jcomdis.2022.106200
Crouch, E., Probst, J. C., Radcliff, E., Bennett, K. J., & McKinney, S. H. (2019). Prevalence of adverse childhood experiences (ACEs) among US children. *Child Abuse & Neglect, 92*, 209–218. https://doi.org/10.1016/j.chiabu.2019.04.010
Crouch, E., Radcliff, E., Brown, M. J., & Hung, P. (2023). Association between positive childhood experiences and childhood flourishing among US children. *Journal of Developmental and Behavioral Pediatrics, 44*(4), e255–e262. https://doi.org/10.1097/dbp.0000000000001181
Dang, K., Bent, S., Lawton, B., Warren, T., Widjaja, F., McDonald, M. G., Breard, M., O'Keefe, W., & Hendren, R. L. (2017). Integrating autism care through a school-based intervention model: A pilot study. *Journal of Clinical Medicine, 6*(10). https://doi.org/10.3390/jcm6100097
Dawes, D. E., Kirby, R., Dunlap, N., & Valle, M. (2022). An overview of maternal and child health history: A political determinants of health perspective. In R. S. Kirby & S. Verbiest (Eds.), *Kotch's maternal and child health: Problems, programs, and policy in public health* (4th ed., pp. 81–96). Jones & Bartlett Learning.
Dawson, A. E., LaMotte, J. E., & Bignall, O. N. R., 2nd. (2022). Acknowledging socioecological systems to address the systemic racial disparities in children with kidney disease. *Journal of the American Society of Nephrology, 33*(10), 1820–1822. https://doi.org/10.1681/asn.2022040428
Education for All Handicapped Children Act of 1975, 89 Stat. 773.
Elder, G. H. J. (2006). Life course perspective. In G. Ritzer (Ed.), *The Blackwell encyclopedia of sociology* (pp. 2634–2639). Blackwell.

El-Hattab, A. W., Almannai, M., & Sutton, V. R. (2018). Newborn screening: History, current status, and future directions. *Pediatric Clinics, 65*(2), 389–405.

Family Voices. (2025). *Family-Centered Care.* Retrieved July 2, 2025 from https://familyvoices.org/familycenteredcare/

Forsythe, J. S. (1939). Legislative history of the Fair Labor Standards Act. *Law and Contemporary Problems, 6*, 464. Available at: https://heinonline.org/HOL/LandingPage?handle=hein.journals/lcp6&div=43&id=&page=

Gernsbacher, M. A., Raimond, A. R., Balinghasay, M. T., & Boston, J. S. (2016). "Special needs" is an ineffective euphemism. *Cognitive Research: Principles and Implications, 1*(1), 29. https://doi.org/10.1186/s41235-016-0025-4

Ghandour, R. M., Jones, J. R., Lebrun-Harris, L. A., Minnaert, J., Blumberg, S. J., Fields, J., Bethell, C., & Kogan, M. D. (2018). The design and implementation of the 2016 National Survey of Children's Health. *Maternal and Child Health Journal, 22*(8), 1093–1102. https://doi.org/10.1007/s10995-018-2526-x

Ghandour, R. M., Hirai, A. H., & Kenney, M. K. (2022). Children and youth with special health care needs: A profile. *Pediatrics, 149*(Supplement 7). https://doi.org/10.1542/peds.2021-056150D

Grech, L. B., Koller, D., & Olley, A. (2023). Furthering the person-first versus identity-first language debate. *Australian Psychologist, 58*(4), 223–232.

Guralnick, M. J. (2011). Why early intervention works: A systems perspective. *Infants and Young Children, 24*(1), 6–28. https://doi.org/10.1097/IYC.0b013e3182002cfe

Guralnick, M. J. (2020). Applying the developmental systems approach to inclusive community-based early intervention programs: Process and practice. *Infants and Young Children, 33*(3), 173–183. https://doi.org/10.1097/IYC.0000000000000167

Halfon, N., Russ, S. A., & Counts, N. Z. (2024). Time for a kids progress administration: US Department of the Treasury stepping up. *JAMA Pediatrics, 178*(7), 643–644.

Hall, M. C. (2019). Critical disability theory. Retrieved from https://plato.stanford.edu/archives/win2019/entries/disability-critical/

Health Resources & Services Administration. (n.d.). Maternal, Infant, and Early Childhood Home Visiting (MIECHV) Program. Retrieved June 21, 2025 from https://mchb.hrsa.gov/programs-impact/maternal-infant-early-childhood-home-visiting-miechv-program

Hodapp, R. M. (2007). Families of persons with Down syndrome: New perspectives, findings, and research and service needs. *Mental Retardation and Developmental Disabilities Research Reviews, 13*(3), 279–287. https://doi.org/10.1002/mrdd.20160

Houtrow, A., Martin, A. J., Harris, D., Cejas, D., Hutson, R., Mazloomdoost, Y., & Agrawal, R. K. (2022). Health equity for children and youth with special health care needs: A vision for the future. *Pediatrics, 149*(Suppl 7). https://doi.org/10.1542/peds.2021-056150F

Hsu, C., Gray, M. F., Murray, L., Abraham, M., Nickel, W., Sweeney, J. M., Frosch, D. L., Mroz, T. M., Ehrlich, K., Johnson, B., & Reid, R. J. (2019). Actions and processes that patients, family members, and physicians associate with patient- and family-centered care. *BMC Family Practice, 20*(1), 35. https://doi.org/10.1186/s12875-019-0918-7

Huang, L., Freed, G. L., & Dalziel, K. (2020). Children with special health care needs: How special are their health care needs? *Academic Pediatrics, 20*(8), 1109–1115. https://doi.org/10.1016/j.acap.2020.01.007

Huang, C. X., Halfon, N., Sastry, N., Chung, P. J., & Schickedanz, A. (2023). Positive childhood experiences and adult health outcomes. *Pediatrics, 152*(1), e2022060951. https://doi.org/10.1542/peds.2022-060951

Hyman, S. L., Levy, S. E., Myers, S. M., & Council on Children with Disabilities, & Section on Developmental and Behavioral Pediatrics. (2020). Identification, evaluation, and management of children with autism spectrum disorder. *Pediatrics, 145*(1), e20193447. https://doi.org/10.1542/peds.2019-3447

Individuals with Disabilities Education Improvement Act (IDEA) of 2004, Public Law 446, U.S. Statutes at Large 118 (2004): 2647–2808. https://www.govinfo.gov/app/details/STATUTE-118/STATUTE-118-Pg2647

Irving, C., Basu, A., Richmond, S., Burn, J., & Wren, C. (2008). Twenty-year trends in prevalence and survival of Down syndrome. *European Journal of Human Genetics, 16*(11), 1336–1340. https://doi.org/10.1038/ejhg.2008.122

Johnson, K. (2011). New evidence on program impact can guide implementation of federal home visiting program. *Archives of Pediatric & Adolescent Medicine, 165*(3), 278–279. https://doi.org/10.1001/archpediatrics.2010.220

Johnson, B., Abraham, M., Conway, J., Simmons, L., Edgman-Levitan, S., Sodomka, P., Schlucter, J., & Ford, D. (2008). *Partnering with Patients and Families to design a Patient- and Family-Centered health Care system: Recommendations and Promising Practices.* www.ipfcc.org

Jones Harden, B., Chazan-Cohen, R., Raikes, H., & Vogel, C. (2012). Early Head Start home visitation: The role of implementation in bolstering program benefits. *Journal of Community Psychology, 40*(4), 438–455. https://doi.org/10.1002/jcop.20525

Kan, K., Gupta, R., Davis, M. M., Heard-Garris, N., & Garfield, C. (2020). Adverse experiences and special health care needs among children. *Maternal and Child Health Journal, 24*(5), 552–560. https://doi.org/10.1007/s10995-020-02874-x

Kart, A., & Kart, M. (2021). Academic and social effects of inclusion on students without disabilities: A review of the literature. *Education Sciences, 11*(1), 16. https://doi.org/10.3390/educsci11010016

Kempe, C. H., Silverman, F. N., Steele, B. F., Droegemueller, W., & Silver, H. K. (1962). The battered-child syndrome. *Journal of the American Medical Association, 181*(1), 17–24. https://doi.org/10.1001/jama.1962.03050270019004

Kikuhara, M., Hirakami, K., Tamasaki, A., Maegaki, Y., & Hanaki, K. (2021). The process by which mothers of children with special healthcare needs evolve their connections with the community. *Nursing and Health Sciences, 23*(4), 957–966. https://doi.org/10.1111/nhs.12887

Kindratt, T. B., Lark, P., Ray, M., & Brannon, G. E. (2022). Disparities in patient- and family-centered care among children with health conditions. *Journal of Patient Experience, 9*, 23743735221092494. https://doi.org/10.1177/23743735221092494

Kogan, M. D., Strickland, B. B., Blumberg, S. J., Singh, G. K., Perrin, J. M., & van Dyck, P. C. (2008). A national profile of the health care experiences and family impact of autism spectrum disorder among children in the United States, 2005–2006 [Article]. *Pediatrics, 122*(6), e1149–e1158. https://doi.org/10.1542/peds.2008-1057

Kotch, J. (2013). *Maternal and child health: Programs, problems, and policy in public health.* Jones & Bartlett Learning. https://books.google.com/books?id=VtmKhxCleWwC

Kouo, J. L., Kouo, T. S., & Gallogly, J. (2022). Brief report: The experiences of families of children with an Autism Spectrum Disorder when seeking patient-and family-centered care. *Journal of Autism and Developmental Disorders, 52*(9), 4172–4180. https://doi.org/10.1007/s10803-021-05272-6

Kuh, D., & Ben-Shlomo, Y. (1997). Introduction. In *A life course approach to chronic disease epidemiology* (1st ed., pp. 3–16). Oxford University Press.

Kuo, D. Z., Rodgers, R. C., Beers, N. S., McLellan, S. E., & Nguyen, T. K. (2022). Access to services for children and youth with special health care needs and their families: Concepts and considerations for an integrated systems redesign. *Pediatrics, 149*(S1-S7), e2021056150H. https://doi.org/10.1542/peds.2021-056150H

Lee, K., & Luellen, J. L. (2021). Long-term Head Start impacts on cognitive outcomes for children with disabilities. *Families in Society: Journal of Contemporary Social Services, 102*(1), 104–118. https://doi.org/10.1177/1044389420926131

Lichstein, J. C., Ghandour, R. M., & Mann, M. Y. (2018). Access to the medical home among children with and without special health care needs. *Pediatrics, 142*(6), e20181795. https://doi.org/10.1542/peds.2018-1795

Lohnmann, M. J., Hovey, K. A., & Gauvreau, A. N. (2018). Using a universal design for learning framework to enhance engagement in the early childhood classroom. *Journal of Special Education Apprenticeship, 7*(2). https://doi.org/10.58729/2167-3454.1072

Lollar, D. J., & Crews, J. E. (2003). Redefining the role of public health in disability. *Annual Review of Public Health, 24*(1), 195–208. https://doi.org/10.1146/annurev.publhealth.24.100901.140844

Lu, M. C., & Halfon, N. (2003). Racial and ethnic disparities in birth outcomes: A life-course perspective. *Maternal and Child Health Journal, 7*(1), 13–30. https://doi.org/10.1023/A:1022537516969

Lubetsky, M. J., Handen, B. L., Lubetsky, M., & McGonigle, J. J. (2014). Systems of care for individuals with autism spectrum disorder and serious behavioral disturbance through the lifespan. *Child and Adolescent Psychiatric Clinics of North America, 23*(1), 97–110. https://doi.org/10.1016/j.chc.2013.08.004

Mahnke, C. B. (2000). The growth and development of a specialty: The history of pediatrics. *Clinical Pediatrics, 39*(12), 705–714. https://doi.org/10.1177/000992280003901204

Masten, A. S. (2018). Resilience theory and research on children and families: Past, present, and promise. *Journal of Family Theory & Review, 10*(1), 12–31. https://doi.org/10.1111/jftr.12255

Masten, A. S., & Cicchetti, D. (2016). Resilience in development: Progress and transformation. In D. Cicchetti (Ed.), *Developmental psychopathology: Risk, resilience, and intervention* (3rd ed., pp. 271–333). Wiley. https://doi.org/10.1002/9781119125556.devpsy406

McConkey, R., Slater, P., Dubois, L., Shellard, A., & Smith, A. (2022). Engagement with Special Olympics by the general public in 17 countries world-wide. *Sport in Society, 25*(9), 1766–1777. https://doi.org/10.1080/17430437.2020.1830971

McDonald, K. E., & Raymaker, D. M. (2013). Paradigm shifts in disability and health: Toward more ethical public health research. *American Journal of Public Health, 103*(12), 2165–2173. https://doi.org/10.2105/AJPH.2013.301286

McKelvey, L. M., Whiteside-Mansell, L., Conners-Burrow, N. A., Swindle, T., & Fitzgerald, S. (2016). Assessing adverse experiences from infancy through early childhood in home visiting programs. *Child Abuse & Neglect, 51*, 295–302.

McPherson, M., Arango, P., Fox, H., Lauver, C., McManus, M., Newacheck, P. W., Perrin, J. M., Shonkoff, J. P., & Strickland, B. (1998). A new definition of children with special health care needs. *Pediatrics, 102*(1 Pt 1), 137–140. https://doi.org/10.1542/peds.102.1.137

Mendel, P., Chen, E. K., Green, H. D., Armstrong, C., Timbie, J. W., Kress, A. M., Friedberg, M. W., & Kahn, K. L. (2018). Pathways to medical home recognition: A qualitative comparative analysis of the PCMH transformation process. *Health Services Research, 53*(4), 2523–2546. https://doi.org/10.1111/1475-6773.12803

Mestre, T. D., Lopes, M. J., Mestre, D. M., Ferreira, R. F., Costa, A. P., & Caldeira, E. V. (2024). Impact of family-centered care in families with children with intellectual disability: A systematic review. *Heliyon, 10*(7), e28241. https://doi.org/10.1016/j.heliyon.2024.e28241

Ming, X., Hashim, A., Fleishman, S., West, T., Kang, N., Chen, X., & Zimmerman-Bier, B. (2011). Access to specialty care in autism spectrum disorders-a pilot study of referral source. *BMC Health Services Research, 11*(1), 99. https://doi.org/10.1186/1472-6963-11-99

Morgan, P. L., Hu, E. H., Woods, A. D., Gloski, C. A., & Wang, Y. (2022). Disparities in family-centered care among US children and youth with special health care needs. *The Journal of Pediatrics*. https://doi.org/10.1016/j.jpeds.2022.09.024

Myśliwiec, A., & Damentko, M. (2015). Global initiative of the Special Olympics movement for people with intellectual disabilities. *Journal of Human Kinetics, 45*(1), 253–259. https://doi.org/10.1515/hukin-2015-0026

Nugent, J., Gorman, G., & Erdie-Lalena, C. R. (2018). Disparities in access to healthcare transition services for adolescents with Down syndrome. *Journal of Pediatrics, 197*, 214–220. https://doi.org/10.1016/j.jpeds.2018.01.072

Oliver, M. (1990). *The politics of disablement*. Macmillan Education UK.

Oliver, M. (2013). The social model of disability: Thirty years on. *Disability & Society, 28*(7), 1024–1026. https://doi.org/10.1080/09687599.2013.818773

Olson, M. (1965). *Logic of collective action: Public goods and the theory of groups*. Harvard University Press.

Ornstein, M. T., & Caruso, C. C. (2024). The social ecology of caregiving: Applying the Social–Ecological Model across the life course. *International Journal of Environmental Research and Public Health, 21*(1), 119. https://doi.org/10.3390/ijerph21010119

Osterman, M., Hamilton, B., Martin, J. A., Driscoll, A. K., & Valenzuela, C. P. (2021). Births: Final data for 2020. *National Vital Statistics Reports, 70*(17), 1–50.

Ostrom, E. (1990). *Governing the commons: The evolution of institutions for collective action.* Cambridge University Press. https://doi.org/10.1017/CBO9780511807763

Pennington, J. R., Oglesby, W. H., & Alemagno, S. (2021). Impact of social capital on the availability of health care services. *Population Health Management, 24*(3), 369–375. https://doi.org/10.1089/pop.2020.0142

Perrin, E. C., Newacheck, P., Pless, I. B., Drotar, D., Gortmaker, S. L., Leventhal, J., Perrin, J. M., Stein, R. E., Walker, D. K., & Weitzman, M. (1993). Issues involved in the definition and classification of chronic health conditions. *Pediatrics, 91*(4), 787–793.

Peters, C. P. (2006). *EPSDT: Medicaid's critical but controversial benefits program for children.* National Health Policy Forum. Paper 174.Retrieved June 21, 2025 from https://hsrc.himmelfarb.gwu.edu/sphhs_centers_nhpf/174

Procknow, G., Rocco, T. S., & Munn, S. L. (2017). (Dis)Ableing notions of authentic leadership through the lens of critical disability theory. *Advances in Developing Human Resources, 19*(4), 362–377. https://doi.org/10.1177/1523422317728732

Ralston, K., Newman, C., Clauson, A., Guthrie, J., & Buzby, J. (2008). *The National School Lunch Program: Background, trends, and issues.* Economic Research Report Number 61. US Department of Agriculture.

Rast, J., Newschaffer, C., Turchi, R., & Plumb, J. (2021). Health service and functional measures of benefit of a medical home in children with Autism. *Maternal and Child Health Journal, 25*(7), 1156–1163. https://doi.org/10.1007/s10995-021-03150-2

Rast, J. E., Garfield, T., Ezeh, T. H., & Anderson, K. A. (2024). Mental health, race and ethnicity, and medical home in children with special health care needs. *Children's Health Care, 53*(4), 374–388. https://doi.org/10.1080/02739615.2023.2212905

Reaume, G. (2014). Understanding critical disability studies. *Canadian Medical Association Journal, 186*(16), 1248–1249. https://doi.org/10.1503/cmaj.141236

Rocco, T. S. (2005). From disability studies to critical race theory: Working towards critical disability theory. Adult Education Research Conference. https://newprairiepress.org/aerc/2005/papers/17/

Russo, J., & Wooley, S. (2020). The implementation of the convention on the rights of persons with disabilities: More than just another reform of psychiatry. *Health and Human Rights, 22*(1), 151–161.

Shi, L., Lee, D. C., Chung, M., Liang, H., Lock, D., & Sripipatana, A. (2017). Patient-centered medical home recognition and clinical performance in U.S. community health centers. *Health Services Research, 52*(3), 984–1004. https://doi.org/10.1111/1475-6773.12523

Simpson, T. E., Condon, E., Price, R. M., Finch, B. K., Sadler, L. S., & Ordway, M. R. (2016). Demystifying infant mental health: What the primary care provider needs to know. *Journal of Pediatric Health Care, 30*(1), 38–48. https://doi.org/10.1016/j.pedhc.2015.09.011

Skotko, B. G., Levine, S. P., Macklin, E. A., & Goldstein, R. D. (2016). Family perspectives about Down syndrome. *American Journal of Medical Genetics. Part A, 170A*(4), 930–941. https://doi.org/10.1002/ajmg.a.37520

Son, E., Moring, N. S., Igdalsky, L., & Parish, S. L. (2018). Navigating the health-care system in community: Perspectives from Asian immigrant parents of children with special health-care needs. *Journal of Child Health Care, 22*(2), 251–268. https://doi.org/10.1177/1367493517753084

Stein Elger, R., Valencia, J., Silva Correia, J., Abdallah, A., Bakour, C., & Kirby, R. S. (2023). The impact of adverse childhood experiences (ACEs) on sleep adequacy for children with special health care needs (CSHCN) in the United States. *Disability and Health Journal, 16*(4), 101498. https://doi.org/10.1016/j.dhjo.2023.101498

Stoltzfus, E. (2009). *The Child Abuse Prevention and Treatment ct (CAPTA): Background, programs, and funding.* Congressional Research Service, 7–5700.

Strickland, B. B., Singh, G. K., Kogan, M. D., Mann, M. Y., van Dyck, P. C., & Newacheck, P. W. (2009). Access to the medical home: New findings from the 2005–2006 National Survey of Children with Special Health Care Needs. *Pediatrics, 123*(6), e996–e1004. https://doi.org/10.1542/peds.2008-2504

Stroul, B. A., & Blau, G. M. (2010). Defining the system of care concept and philosophy: To update or not to update? *Evaluation and Program Planning, 33*(1), 59–62. https://doi.org/10.1016/j.evalprogplan.2009.06.003

Stroul, B. A., & Friedman, R. M. (1986). *A system of care for children and youth with severe emotional disturbances* (Rev. ed). CASSP Technical Assistance Center, Center for Child Health and Mental Health Policy, Georgetown University Child Development Center. https://www.ojp.gov/pdffiles1/Digitization/125081NCJRS.pdf

Stroul, B., Blau, G., & Friedman, R. (2010). *Updating the system of care concept and philosophy.* Georgetown University Center for Child and Human Development, National Technical Assistance Center for Children's Mental Health. https://www.isbe.net/Documents/soc-brief-2010.pdf

Stroul, B., Goldman, S., Pires, S., & Manteuffel, B. (2012). *Expanding systems of care: Improving the lives of children, youth, and families.* Georgetown University Center for Child and Human Development, National Technical Assistance Center for Children's Mental Health. https://gucchd.georgetown.edu/products/SOC%20Results%205-7-12.pdf

Turgeon, S., Turgeon, J., & Morin, D. (2023). Coaching Special Olympics: A scoping review. *International Journal of Sports Science & Coaching, 18*(1), 304–323. https://doi.org/10.1177/17479541221134338

United Nations. (1989). Convention on the Rights of the Child. *Treaty Series, 1577*, 3.

United Nations. (2006). Convention on the Rights of Persons with Disabilities. *Treaty Series, 2515*, 3.

United States Maternal and Child Health Bureau. (2010). *Rethinking MCH: The life course model as an organizing framework: Concept paper.* U.S. Department of Health and Human Services, Health Resources and Services Administration, Maternal and Child Health Bureau. https://books.google.com/books?id=qIlfywAACAAJ

US Department of Agriculture. (2024). Legislative history of breastfeeding promotion requirements in WIC. Retrieved June 21, 2025 from https://www.fns.usda.gov/wic/legislative-history-breastfeeding-promotion-requirements-wic

US DHHS. (n.d.). Administration for Children and Families OHS Fact Sheet. Available at https://acf.gov/ohs/comms-fact-sheet/office-head-start

Vanegas, S. B., & Abdelrahim, R. (2016). Characterizing the systems of support for families of children with disabilities: A review of the literature. *Journal of Family Social Work, 19*(4), 286–327. https://doi.org/10.1080/10522158.2016.1218399

Vicente, D., Venegas, M., Coker, T. R., & Guerrero, A. D. (2022). Promoting child development during the COVID-19 Pandemic: Parental perceptions of Tele-Home Visits in Early Head Start Programs. *Maternal and Child Health Journal, 26*(12), 2496–2505. https://doi.org/10.1007/s10995-022-03520-4

Warren, M. D., McLellan, S. E., Mann, M. Y., Scott, J. A., & Brown, T. W. (2022). Progress, persistence, and hope: Building a system of services for CYSHCN and their families. *Pediatrics, 149*(Suppl 7). https://doi.org/10.1542/peds.2021-056150E

Watkinson, M. D., Ehlenbach, M., Chung, P. J., Kelly, M., Werner, N., Jolliff, A., Katz, B., Marleau, H., Nacht, C. L., Warner, G., & Coller, R. J. (2023). Interventions in the home and community for medically complex children: A systematic review. *Pediatrics, 151*(5). https://doi.org/10.1542/peds.2022-058352

Williams, N. J., Beauchemin, J., Giuntini, G., Griffis, J., & Mo, Y. (2021). Psychometric evaluation of a pragmatic measure for assessing adherence to system of care principles in behavioral health service interactions. *Journal of Emotional and Behavioral Disorders, 30*(3), 221–234. https://doi.org/10.1177/10634266211028204

Willits, K. A., Platonova, E. A., Nies, M. A., Racine, E. F., Troutman, M. L., & Harris, H. L. (2013). Medical home and pediatric primary care utilization among children with special health care needs. *Journal of Pediatric Health Care, 27*(3), 202–208. https://doi.org/10.1016/j.pedhc.2011.11.004

Chapter 12
Functioning in Key Contexts for Children with Developmental Disabilities and Illnesses and Directions for Future Research

Tina L. Stanton-Chapman and Laura Nabors

Abstract This chapter synthesizes key themes from the book, emphasizing the remarkable resilience and adaptability of children with developmental disabilities and chronic illnesses. Resilience is fostered when challenges are reframed as opportunities for individualized support tailored to each child's strengths. Effective interventions prioritize building teacher self-efficacy, which shapes inclusive classroom environments and leads to positive student outcomes through structured supports and accommodations. Teacher coaching, mentorship, and targeted interventions are highlighted as evidence-based approaches, especially when customized for different subgroups. The chapter stresses the importance of family-centered practices, empowering caregivers as active partners and facilitating collaboration among educators, health professionals, parents, and children. Comprehensive parent support programs build coping skills, reduce isolation, and support school participation during medical episodes. Adopting a systems of care approach rooted in ecological theory, the chapter advocates for integrating community supports and assessing risk and resilience across various contexts. Future research is needed to refine and optimize these supports further.

Keywords Intervention · Resilience · Methods · Developmental disabilities · Chronic illnesses

At the conclusion of an edited book, one question that readers often ask is, *what is the overall point or main message that the authors wish to make?* Often, there are

T. L. Stanton-Chapman (✉)
Elementary Education and Human Development, College of Education, Criminal Justice, Human Services, and Information Technology, University of Cincinnati, Cincinnati, OH, USA
e-mail: stantot@ucmail.uc.edu

L. Nabors
School of Human Services, University of Cincinnati, Cincinnati, OH, USA

L. Nabors and T. Stanton-Chapman (eds.), *Developmental Disabilities and Chronic Illness in Young Children*, Springer Series on Child and Family Studies,
https://doi.org/10.1007/978-3-032-08523-8_12

multiple main points. In the current book, there are several take-home points which are divided into two categories: general and specific. The general points refer to the principles upon which this book is based. The specific points are the basic findings within each chapter about developmental disabilities and chronic illnesses in young children.

General Points

Resilience

Reading across the chapters in this edited book, it is clear that children with developmental disabilities or chronic illnesses are resilient. They possess a remarkable capacity to cope, learn, and grow from their challenges. Resilience is formally defined as an individual's ability to anticipate, adapt, and adjust to difficulties in one's life (Ungar, 2018). Throughout this book, the authors' consistently offered the message that the disabilities and chronic illnesses experienced by children should not be considered as deficits but rather as opportunities to offer appropriate supports that focus on the children's abilities. Indeed, when adults provide consistent supports, positive reinforcement, and environmental contexts that adapt to the children's abilities, successes within this population are discovered.

Intervention

Educational and medical interventions provide children with the supports needed to acquire the skills taught in a given environmental context (Lestrud, 2013). Interventions help children overcome barriers in learning, develop new skills, and improve academic and social performance. In order to determine which intervention should be used with a child, appropriate evaluations and assessments are needed (Rossmann et al., 2023). The interventions described within this book are examples of best practices that are aimed at improving the outcomes for children with developmental disabilities or chronic illnesses. The sooner these interventions are put in place, the sooner the children can experience success in academic, peer, and family endeavors.

Methods and Approaches

The research described across the chapters utilizes a variety of methods and approaches to the study of developmental disabilities and chronic illnesses. These methods and approaches range from randomized controlled trials to rigorous qualitative studies. Each approach provides a window through which to view the developing child. One window alone, however, does not provide a complete picture of evidence-based practices for children with developmental disabilities or chronic illnesses. The collection of methods and approaches is more likely to provide a more complete understanding of what works and under what conditions the methods and approaches work. In general, developmental conclusions are most evident when they are based on converging evidence from several types of studies and replicated across multiple populations.

Specific Points

Faithful Inclusion

Children with developmental disabilities or chronic illnesses often are not included or supported in the faith community. Prior research (e.g., Miller-Perrin & Mancuso, 2014) highlights the vital role faith communities offer to individuals, in general, such as offering support, providing a sense of community, and building spiritual growth. As reported in Chap. 2, faith communities hold great potential as places of inclusion and belonging for children with developmental disabilities or chronic illnesses and their families. Faith communities have been found to offer families sources of strength and resilience, connect them to much-needed practical, emotional, spiritual, and personal supports, and contribute to their overall wellbeing. Interventions targeting faith communities are not only critical for the inclusion of children with disabilities but are crucial in the training of faith communities so they are better prepared to offer a more inclusive environment within their faith community. Intervention strategies include reflection, proactively planning for children with developmental disabilities or chronic illnesses and their families, inviting families who have children with developmental disabilities or chronic illnesses to their congregation, teaching other families strategies on how to support and include families with children with developmental disabilities, and advocating for inclusion throughout the local community. While more research is needed within faith communities, initial data does offer support for this type of work. Additionally, research on the role of support in different types of faith-based communities, and the types of support they offer, will provide new information to guide the field.

Inclusion within School Settings

Teacher self-efficacy refers to a teacher's belief in their ability to successfully cope with classroom tasks, obligations, and challenges related to their professional role

(Barni et al., 2019). As indicated in Chap. 3, a teacher's self-efficacy influences children's experiences in the classroom environment, teacher-student relationships, academic achievement, and children's social and behavioral outcomes. Teachers, who have higher self-efficacy, tend to provide a structured learning environment with appropriate accommodations and supports for children with developmental disabilities or chronic illnesses. Two forms of intervention help promote positive outcomes in children with developmental disabilities or chronic illnesses—teacher coaching and mentoring and child intervention. Teacher coaching and mentoring not only assists teachers with any self-doubt but it has the potential to influence their ability to create a supportive environment for students of all abilities. Child interventions are evidence-based supports provided to children by teachers to support their inclusion in the least restrictive environment. Such interventions are highly influential in positive child outcomes. Research on what works for whom, specifying what supports work for what types of special needs for children of different ages and ethnic groups will provide specialized knowledge to tailor interventions to child needs. Also, finding ways to involve parents in research—to gain more knowledge about their perceptions of education and needs for their child will continue to inform the field.

Playground Inclusion

Social participation refers to an individual's ability to engage with the physical environment and interact with others who are in that environment at the same time (Chap. 4). Studies examining the social participation of children with disabilities on playgrounds reported one of three options: (a) their child with a disability stayed home while other family members participated in outdoor play, (b) the family drove over 30-min from their home to locate more inclusive playground facilities, and/or (c) the family participated in activities at home (e.g., board games). This research highlighted (a) the need for a playground environment that meets the needs of *all* children, (b) the segregation that takes place on a playground between children with and without disabilities, and (c) the lack of interest in accessible playgrounds in children of all abilities. A universal playground is one that addresses the exclusion of children with developmental disabilities or chronic illnesses on the playground setting. Universal playgrounds are playgrounds in which every child regardless of gender, race/ethnicity, age, or ability or disability is welcomed and benefits physically, developmentally, and socially. Research on universal playgrounds shows they are highly effective in building social participation skills in children with developmental disabilities. Designing playgrounds with playground equipment that is proven effective through rigorous research should be seen as central to community playground builds and intervention.

Extracurricular Activity Inclusion

Dymond and Pence (Chap. 5) examine involvement of children with special needs in extracurricular activities, which are those activities which extend beyond the school curriculum. Their chapter highlights how involvement in activities can improve physical, social, and emotional development, with an eye toward designing an environment that facilitates inclusion and the safety of the child with a special need. Involving children in extracurricular activities often involves navigating environmental and safety changes and finding adults to support the child during the activity. However, involvement in extracurricular activities is an important support and service for youth, as indicated by Ayers and coauthors in Chap. 10. There is a range of activities that can work, including sports (which are a more common area for involving young children), social clubs, recreation center activities, art, music (e.g., band), and drama.

Unfortunately, children with special needs may have low rates of participation in extracurricular activities, and low rates of participation may be especially common for children with developmental disabilities (Coster et al., 2013; Kim et al., 2024). Dymond and Pence stress that having a written plan can facilitate involvement, and that including extracurricular activities at school in individual education planning is an avenue for planning for involvement in school-based extracurricular activities. Dymond and Pence reported that support from adults (coaches, parents, other caregivers, teachers) can facilitate inclusion as well as ensuring that children have assistive technologies available to facilitate communication and help them overcome physical limitations during activities (Pence & Dymond, 2016, 2021). Planning for inclusion in extracurricular activities may begin with a search for what is available and then developing a plan for involvement in the activity or activities. Safety monitoring and adjustments for the environment to facilitate inclusion are a key part of planning for successful involvement (Ballard and Dymond, 2018, 2023). Ensuring that medical professionals advise about accommodations and having other health professionals (e.g., physical therapists, occupational therapists, psychologists, special education teachers) provide guidance can improve the success of plans for inclusion. Research on the social, emotional, and physical changes and potentially growth for children involved in different types of activities will improve knowledge in the field. Moreover, learning more about support needs for children with different types of disabilities and illnesses will provide information about what supports are needed for children with different types of special needs—providing information for interventions to guide adults leading extracurricular activities.

Siblings and Children with Developmental Disabilities or Chronic Illnesses

In Chap. 6, Donnelly and Frankovich discuss sibling development (siblings of children with special needs) and their role in the family. These authors also take a systems approach—emphasizing sibling involvement as improving family cohesion. Open communication—facilitated by parents—can improve the sibling experience, role, and family functioning. Parents or caregivers can help siblings and their child with a health condition or developmental disability by fostering open communication, where everyone is sharing and figuring out steps toward positive family adjustment and functioning together, as in most instances, teamwork fosters resilience of the family unit. Siblings experience joy and positive interactions with their brother or sister who has a special healthcare need (Rixon et al., 2025). Siblings often have a caregiving role in their brother or sister's care (Hayden et al., 2023), and open communication helps them to navigate this role and their feelings about it. Siblings may experience a mix of feelings and reactions along with the joy of interacting with their brother or sister. The stressors related to having a sibling with a special healthcare needs can include feelings of isolation, mental health concerns (e.g., depression), caregiving stress, guilt about having a normal developmental course, and loyalty to the sibling and family (Hanvey et al. 2022). As such, it is important to support sibling development, achievements, and need for care and understanding of how to cope with challenges. Understanding what supports both siblings and their brother or sister with a special healthcare need and how they can bond will provide information to bolster the development of siblings and children with special needs. Moreover, the information will provide information to parents and professionals so that they can intervene to strengthen relationships and positive family interactions.

Role of Families

Family-centered practice is an intervention approach which focuses on empowering families by emphasizing strengths, building capacity, and fostering collaboration to promote positive child and family outcomes (Dunst & Trivette, 2014). A focal point of family-centered intervention is the viewpoint that the child is a part of their family and services should be provided within the family unit. Central features of family-centered intervention, as highlighted in Chap. 7, include having caregivers serve as the intervention agent and coaches assisting caregivers as they implement interventions. Together, these central features are designed to build caregivers' capacities in assisting their children with developmental disabilities or chronic illnesses to achieve positive outcomes. Understanding ways to involve the family in determining what works, in terms of adherence to medical regimens and in care of children with developmental disabilities will ensure that interventions are optimized to be successful for the family. Moreover, further research assessing how health professionals engage parents and children will provide knowledge to design interventions to improve interactions between health professionals, parents, and children.

Peer Supports

Chapter 8 presents information on the value of peer support for children with illnesses and neurodiversity. Pallotto and her colleagues discuss the critical nature of peer support in facilitating social development during infancy, toddlerhood, the preschool years and beyond. The impact of positive social support is iatrogenic benefitting the child and family for years (Parker et al., 2015). Young children need family support to ensure peer interactions (Lamb & Bornstein, 2013); therefore, parents may benefit from education about the benefits of peer support. Part of this education can be about the mental health benefits of peer support, and its value as an antidote to depression and anxiety for young children with illnesses, neurodiversity, and special healthcare needs (La Greca et al., 2002; van Harmelen et al., 2016).

Pallotto et al. highlighted the value of assessment to determine the types of support that would be best to promote child growth and development. Some children may benefit from education about social skills, while others can benefit from support groups. Involvement in extracurricular activities can be beneficial for some, while others may need peer buddies to facilitate their involvement at recess at school. When determining what types of peer support are needed, it is critical to consult with medical professionals to understand physical abilities and contraindications for involvement in different types of activities. In schools, discussing social involvement with teachers can facilitate developing plans to promote social skills and interactions with peers. Pallotto et al. also mentioned the value of summer camps and peer buddies in reducing isolation and teaching disease management to children (Christiansen et al., 2015; Martiniuk et al., 2014). Involvement with peers—can be an invaluable boost to social and emotional wellbeing, with planning and understanding of the child's needs in different contexts, such as school and extracurricular activities. Research is needed to determine how peers can serve as buddies and provide support across the aforementioned contexts.

Fostering Resilience During Times of Hospitalization

Chapter 9 addresses services for children during hospitalization and upon re-entry into their home and school. Wazevich and her colleagues stress considering the child's system and providing services where they are needed—to enhance child and family resilience. For instance, peer support programs can facilitate child social development and reduce a sense of isolation related to having an illness, if children need social support, during the hospital stay or afterwards (Lancaster et al., 2023). When children return to the community, they can learn self-care of their illness with peers in support groups as well (Lewis et al., 2016). Wazevich and colleagues report supports that can be provided during hospitalization, including social skills coaching, improving communication skills, and therapy or interventions to promote emotional wellbeing. Educational support through connecting with the school or, if available, attending a hospital school or tutoring is important to support the child. In pilot work, Wazevich and her colleagues discovered that parents often serve as tutors, especially when the child has a good grasp of schoolwork.

Parent support is also emphasized in Chap. 9, and there are interventions to teach parents steps of disease management and care as well as cognitive-behavioral skills and problem-solving to promote child coping with illness and resultant emotional and behavioral problems that can occur (Doupnik et al., 2017). The majority of interventions may be multifaceted, with several components, such as teaching care of the illness as well as providing invaluable ideas for social development and support of the family and the child (Doupnik et al., 2017). Parent support also reduces their sense of isolation and learning from other parents in group settings can provide long-term friendships and support as the family navigates the course of the child's illness. Research is needed to determine how to facilitate schooling when children undergo frequent medical procedures and hospitalizations. Moreover, research on how to engage parents and children in shared decision-making about medical care and the medical regimen, during hospitalization and then after re-integration in the home and school settings will continue to guide interventions and clinical care.

Navigating the Service System

Chapter 10 focuses on child and family navigation of complex service systems for children with disabilities. Ayers and her colleagues comment that successful service delivery is flexible and meets family needs and abilities. We define abilities as being things the family is capable of doing and understands. As such, abilities can be expanded with education and more support to the family and child. To that end, family navigators are one type of guide to guage family needs and abilities, while connecting the child and family to services. Several types of navigators are available, including medical navigators. However, given the need for shared decision–making in all aspects of the child's care and development, and limited time for busy families, we propose that family navigators are one potential solution to care coordination that would emphasize family perspectives and capabilities in terms of alignment with services that the family can access and use to benefit their child's development.

Moreover, in Chap. 10, Ayers and her colleagues stress interaction between medical and educational settings as being critical to optimizing the child's development at school (Kuo et al., 2018). This is a wonderful notion, and the authors build from this model, including collaboration between other therapies and services that will foster child physical, emotional, and academic progress. A family navigator or care navigator is often a "lynch pin" for treatment planning for a child with a disability if many services need to be aligned to contribute to the child's growth, wellbeing, and development. It also remains important to consider barriers families face in accessing multiple systems of services, including language barriers, disability status of parents, and cultural differences (Pankewicz et al., 2020). Care coordination or service coordination is essential, so that providers can learn from each other and scaffold their training to build upon successes in the different medical and educational disciplines. Community supports are also essential to child wellbeing and should be considered as part of the child's service package and needs, rather than as ancillary services (Lanchak et al., 2024). In Chap. 10, Ayers and her colleagues discuss the notion of collaborative partnerships to foster child development and growth, and these partnerships can strengthen child development and the family framework, promoting resilience in child development. Research understanding the nature of "best practices" for collaborative partnerships will provide a blueprint for assisting children and their families. Moreover, understanding how practices vary across different types of disabilities and illnesses will provide specific information to inform interventions and for developing support groups and care navigation that allows for optimal support of children with disabilities and chronic illnesses.

Systems of Care for Children with Special Health Care Needs

Chapter 11 addresses children with special healthcare needs (CSHCN). The authors note that about half of CSHCN do not receive care in a medical home (Coller et al., 2020; Ghandour et al., 2018). Unfortunately, CSHCN are more likely to receive poorer care in health care systems than children who are developing typically (Yu et al., 2021). Advocacy is needed to improve their health care and involve parents and, as needed, extended family in family–centered care to improve health and wellbeing of young children in this vulnerable group. Involving parents in shared decision-making may improve health care for CSHCN, as parents have unique knowledge as primary caregivers administering a great deal of medical care for these children (Baker & Claridge, 2022).

Systems of care approaches can benefit CSHCN—ensuring that the interconnected systems within which children seek services are integrated and communicating with one another to meet child needs. The systems of care model is in many ways consistent with Bronfenbrenner's ecological theory, which stresses that overlapping systems shape child development (Bronfenbrenner, 1977). Assessing both risk and resilience factors within systems of care and other key systems in the child's life (e.g., church, school, playground) can provide guidance for developing interventions to promote social and emotional development of CSHCN. Assessment of the impact of interventions throughout the life course (Elder, 2006), to understand their long-term impact and how they influence turning points in children's lives also will provide knowledge to advance the field.

Future Directions to Improve Child Functioning and Family-Centered Care

The authors have summarized applied research in the field. They highlighted the need for future research with young children with developmental disabilities or chronic illnesses. Research examining the impact of peer support and inclusion in different contexts will provide guidance for involving young children with developmental disabilities and chronic illnesses in different settings. Learning about how peer buddies and adults can facilitate social involvement and child development in these different contexts will provide guidance for interventions. Moreover, chapters highlight the importance of a systems approach and family-centered care in assisting children and their families. Learning about how to involve parents and children in shared decision-making may improve family-centered care and parent and child confidence in being a part of the child's medical care and educational development. Understanding steps for involvement in shared decision-making also will provide ideas for health professionals and educators who work with children with special healthcare needs and their families. Finally, learning about best practices for navigating systems of care and for developing the "best fit" or optimal services to wrap-around or provide for children with special healthcare needs can inform clinical practice and the development and implementation of interventions to help young children in this vulnerable group who often face health disparities. Finally, understanding what works for children who have limited access to services, such as those who reside in poverty, will provide critical information to provide services to those most in need of care.

Throughout the book, the authors described intervention and resilience using multiple approaches and methods. Intervention and resilience are interrelated concepts especially in the context of children with developmental disabilities or chronic illnesses. Interventions can be designed to build resilience in children. Conversely, resilience can inform how one develops interventions which target children with developmental disabilities or chronic illnesses. As seen in each chapter, interventions can be implemented in various contexts (e.g., classroom, home, religious settings, playgrounds) that not only build resilience in young children but also promote positive outcomes in their everyday lives.

References

Baker, K., & Claridge, A. M. (2022). "I have a Ph.D. in my daughter": Mother and child experiences of living with childhood chronic illness. *Journal of Child and Family Studies*, 1–12. Advance online publication. https://doi.org/10.1007/s10826-022-02506-8

Ballard, S. L., & Dymond, S. K. (2018). Inclusive education for secondary-age students with severe disabilities and complex health care needs. *Intellectual and Developmental Disabilities, 56*(6), 427–441. https://doi.org/10.1352/1934-9556-56.6.427

Ballard, S., & Dymond, S. K. (2023). Beliefs about secondary-age students with extensive support needs participating in their health care at school. *Research and Practice for Persons with Severe Disabilities, 48*(2), 92–107.
Barni, D., Danioni, F., & Benevene, P. (2019). Teachers' self-efficacy: The role of personal values and motivations for teaching. *Frontiers in Psychology, 10*, 1645. https://doi.org/10.3389/fpsyg.2019.01645
Bronfenbrenner, U. (1977). Toward an experimental ecology of human development. *American Psychologist, 32*(7), 513–531. https://doi.org/10.1037/0003-066X.32.7.513
Christiansen, H. L., Bingen, K., Hoag, J. A., Karst, J. S., Velázquez-Martin, B., & Barakat, L. P. (2015). Providing children and adolescents opportunities for social interaction as a standard of care in pediatric oncology. *Pediatric Blood & Cancer, 62*(S5). https://doi.org/10.1002/pbc.25774
Coller, R. J., Ahrens, S., Ehlenbach, M. L., Shadman, K. A., Mathur, M., Caldera, K., Chung, P. J., LaRocque, A., Peto, H., Binger, K., Smith, W., & Sheehy, A. (2020). Priorities and outcomes for youth-adult transitions in hospital care: Perspectives of inpatient clinical leaders at US children's hospitals. *Hospital Pediatrics, 10*(9), 774–782. https://doi.org/10.1542/hpeds.2020-0016
Coster, W., Law, M., Bedell, G., Liljenquist, K., Kao, Y. C., Khetani, M., & Teplicky, R. (2013). School participation, supports and barriers of students with and without disabilities. *Child: Care, Health and Development, 39*(4), 535–543. https://doi.org/10.1111/cch.12046
Doupnik, S. K., Hill, D., Palakshappa, D., Worsley, D., Bae, H., Shaik, A., Qiu, M. K., Marsac, M., & Feudtner, C. (2017). Parent coping support interventions during acute pediatric hospitalizations: A meta-analysis. *Pediatrics, 140*(3). https://doi.org/10.1542/peds.2016-4171
Dunst, C. J., & Trivette, C. M. (2014). Capacity-building family-systems intervention practices. In G. H. S. Singer, D. E. Biegel, & P. Conway (Eds.), *Family support and family caregiving across disabilities* (pp. 39–63). Routledge.
Elder, G. H. J. (2006). Life course perspective. In G. Ritzer (Ed.), *The Blackwell encyclopedia of sociology* (pp. 2634–2639). Blackwell.
Ghandour, R. M., Jones, J. R., Lebrun-Harris, L. A., Minnaert, J., Blumberg, S. J., Fields, J., Bethell, C., & Kogan, M. D. (2018). The design and implementation of the 2016 National Survey of Children's Health. *Maternal and Child Health Journal, 22*(8), 1093–1102. https://doi.org/10.1007/s10995-018-2526-x
Hanvey, I., Malovic, A., & Ntontis, E. (2022). Glass children: The lived experiences of siblings of people with a disability or chronic illness. *Journal of Community & Applied Social Psychology, 32*. https://doi.org/10.1002/casp.2602
Hayden, N. K., Hastings, R. P., & Bailey, T. (2023). Behavioural adjustment of children with intellectual disability and their sibling is associated with their sibling relationship quality. *Journal of Intellectual Disability Research, 67*(4), 310–322. https://doi.org/10.1111/jir.13006
Kim, M., Jung, J., & Yun, J. (2024). Prevalence of school-based extracurricular sport and physical activity participation among children with disabilities. *International Journal of Disability, Development and Education, 71*(1), 1–12. https://doi.org/10.1080/1034912X.2022.2060947
Kuo, D. Z., McAllister, J. W., Rossignol, L., Turchi, R. M., & Stille, C. J. (2018). Care coordination for children with medical complexity: Whose care is it, anyway? *Pediatrics, 141*(Supplement_3), S224–S232. https://doi.org/10.1542/peds.2017-1284G
La Greca, A. M., Bearman, K. J., & Moore, H. (2002). Peer relations of youth with pediatric conditions and health risks: Promoting social support and healthy lifestyles. *Journal of Developmental & Behavioral Pediatrics, 23*(4), 271.
Lamb, M. E., & Bornstein, M. H. (2013). *Social and personality development: An advanced textbook*. Taylor and Francis.
Lancaster, K., Bhopti, A., Kern, M. L., Taylor, R., Janson, A., & Harding, K. (2023). Effectiveness of peer support programmes for improving well-being and quality of life in parents/carers of children with disability or chronic illness: A systematic review. *Child: Care, Health and Development, 49*(3), 485–496. https://doi.org/10.1111/cch.13063

Lanchak, E. R., Carter, E. W., & McMillan, E. D. (2024). "You don't know what you don't know": Parent perspectives on navigating disability-related information and resources. *Intellectual and Developmental Disabilities, 62*(6), 459–473. https://doi.org/10.1352/1934-9556-62.6.459

Lestrud, M. (2013). Educational interventions. In F. R. Volkmar (Ed.), *Encyclopedia of autism spectrum disorders* (pp. 1061–1062). Springer. https://doi.org/10.1007/978-1-4419-1698-3_1457

Lewis, P., Klineberg, E., Towns, S., Moore, K., & Steinbeck, K. (2016). The effects of introducing peer support to young people with a chronic illness. *Journal of Child and Family Studies, 25*, 2541–2553. https://doi.org/10.1007/s10826-016-0427-4

Martiniuk, A., Silva, M., Amylon, M., & Barr, R. (2014). Camp programs for children with cancer and their families: Review of research progress over the past decade. *Pediatric Blood & Cancer, 61*(5), 778–787. https://doi.org/10.1002/pbc.24912

Miller-Perrin, C., & Mancuso, E. K. (2014). Faith and community. In C. Miller-Perrin & E. K. Mancuso (Eds.), *Faith from a positive psychology perspective* (pp. 183–217). Springer.

Pankewicz, A., Davis, R. K., Kim, J., Antonelli, R., Rosenberg, H., Berhane, Z., & Turchi, R. M. (2020). Children with special needs: Social determinants of health and care coordination. *Clinical Pediatrics, 59*(13), 1161–1168. https://doi.org/10.1177/0009922820941206

Parker, J. G., Rubin, K. H., Erath, S. A., Wojslawowicz, J. C., & Buskirk, A. A. (2015). Peer relationships, child development, and adjustment: A developmental psychopathology perspective. In D. Cicchetti & D. J. Cohen (Eds.), *Developmental psychopathology* (1st ed., pp. 419–493). Wiley. https://doi.org/10.1002/9780470939383.ch12

Pence, A. R., & Dymond, S. K. (2016). Teachers' beliefs about the participation of students with severe disabilities in school clubs. *Research and Practice for Persons with Severe Disabilities, 41*(1), 52–68. https://doi.org/10.1177/1540796915626009

Pence, A. R., & Dymond, S. K. (2021). The participation of secondary students with severe disabilities in school clubs. *Intellectual and Developmental Disabilities, 59*(4), 335–351. https://doi.org/10.1352/1934-9556-59.4.335

Rixon, L., Hastings, R. P., & Kovshoff, H. (2025). 'It feels very weird and normal at the same time': Sibling perceptions of their relationships with an autistic brother of sister with complex care needs. *Journal of Applied Research in Intellectual Disabilities, 38*(1). https://doi.org/10.1111/jar.70009

Rossmann, C., Krnel, S. R., Kylänen, M., Lewtak, K., Tortone, C., Ragazzoni, P., et al. (2023). Health promotion and disease prevention registries in the EU: A cross country comparison. *Archives of Public Health, 81*, 85. https://doi.org/10.1186/s13690-023-01097-0

Ungar, M. (2018). Systemic resilience: Principles and processes for a science of change in contexts of adversity. *Ecology and Society, 23*(4), 34. https://doi.org/10.5751/ES-10385-230434

van Harmelen, A. L., Gibson, J. L., St. Clair, J. C., Owens, M., Brodbeck, J., Dunn, V., Lewis, G.,... & Goodyer, I. M. (2016). Friendships and family support reduce subsequent depressive symptoms in at-risk adolescents. *PLoS ONE, 11*(5), Article e0153715. https://doi.org/10.1371/journal.pone.0153715

Yu, J. A., McKernan, G., Hagerman, T., Schenker, Y., & Houtrow, A. (2021). Identifying children with medical complexity from the national survey of children's health combined 2016–17 data set. *Hospital Pediatrics, 11*(2), 192–197. https://doi.org/10.1542/hpeds.2020-0180

Index

L. Nabors and T. Stanton-Chapman (eds.), *Developmental Disabilities and Chronic Illness in Young Children*, Springer Series on Child and Family Studies,
https://doi.org/10.1007/978-3-032-08523-8

MIX
Papier aus verantwortungsvollen Quellen
Paper from responsible sources
FSC® C105338

If you have any concerns about our products,
you can contact us on
ProductSafety@springernature.com

In case Publisher is established outside the EU,
the EU authorized representative is:
Springer Nature Customer Service Center GmbH
Europaplatz 3, 69115 Heidelberg, Germany

Printed by Libri Plureos GmbH
in Hamburg, Germany